Chair Yoga for Seniors Over 60

for Aches & Pains

Chair Yoga for Seniors Over 60

for Aches & Pains

Improve Mobility and Enhance Flexibility in 10 Minutes a Day

David Anthonie

Zen Over 60

*To those embracing the journey of Zen Over 60—
discovering magic in movement
and strength in simplicity.*

*May fitness renew your energy,
restore your flexibility,
and set you free.*

*May an active life bring you
hope, health, and healing.*

Contents

Chair Yoga for Seniors Over 60

for Aches & Pains

"Zen is discovering

power in the present—

empowerment in practice."

— David Anthonie

Introduction

Are you tired of waking up with aches and pains that limit your ability to enjoy the day? Do you find it difficult to bend down, reach for objects, or simply move comfortably? Are you worried about losing your independence or missing out on activities you love because of stiffness and limitations? You're not alone.

Imagine tapping into a source of energy and healing practiced for centuries. This book is your key to unlocking that potential through chair yoga. Rediscover the magic of movement, experience relief from aches and pains, and reclaim your independence —joining millions who have already transformed their lives.

Picture yourself rising in the morning without aches, or standing up from your favorite chair with ease—no stiffness, no pain, just smooth, easy movement. Imagine effortlessly picking up your grandchild or confidently getting down to the floor and back up without a second thought. This is the life-changing power of chair yoga—a powerful practice that helps you relieve aches and pains, improve mobility, and enhance flexibility in 10 minutes a day.

However, many people face daily challenges with stiffness, tension, and aches that make everyday activities harder to enjoy. This can lead to them avoiding their favorite pastimes or feeling frustrated when their body doesn't move like it did before. But age doesn't have to stop you from living an active life. With the right approach—like chair yoga—anyone can experience renewed energy and freedom in their body.

Chair yoga is uniquely accessible and effective for older adults. It combines the benefits of traditional yoga with the comfort and support of a chair, making it gentle on the joints and adaptable to individual needs. "I used to struggle with back pain and stiffness," says Helen, 72. "But after just a few weeks of chair yoga, I feel more flexible and have more energy than I have in years."

The principles of chair yoga are a proven method that has helped millions of people around the world improve their mobility, reduce pain, and enhance their quality of life. "Chair yoga gave me back my independence," says Robert, 68. "I can move with confidence and enjoy my life without worrying about aches and pains." Like many, Robert's life has been transformed by this healing practice. Their stories demonstrate the power of this approach to improve wellness at any age. With it, you can experience a wide range of benefits, including:

- **Relief from Aches and Pains:** Targeted exercises can soothe discomfort in your back, hips, knees, shoulders, and more.

- **Improved Mobility and Flexibility:** Increased range of motion and flexibility can make everyday activities easier and more enjoyable.

- **Enhanced Balance and Coordination:** Improved balance can help prevent falls and injuries, keeping you active and independent.

- **Increased Energy and Strength:** Chair yoga revitalizes your body and mind, helping you feel refreshed and ready to enjoy each day.

- **Reduced Stress and Anxiety:** Gentle movements and mindful breathing help calm your mind and bring a sense of well-being.

- **Improved Mental Clarity and Focus:** Chair yoga can enhance cognitive function, helping you stay sharp and engaged.

In this book, we'll guide you step-by-step through a series of chair yoga exercises designed specifically for seniors over 60. Each movement is explained in clear, everyday language—no jargon or technical terms— so nobody feels left out. Whether you're new to chair yoga or have some experience, this powerful practice offers benefits that everyone can access. Here's a glimpse of what you'll find in the chapters ahead:

- **Clear Images:** Large, easy-to-understand illustrations.

- **Simple Instructions:** Concise, easy-to-follow instructions.

- **Breathing Guides:** Breathing tips to enhance each movement.

- **Modification Guides:** Variations to adapt the exercises to your needs.

- **Safety Guides:** Tips to ensure you practice safely and with confidence.

- **Benefits Guide:** Detailed descriptions of the benefits of each exercise.

- **7-Day Challenge:** Start with a short challenge to kickstart your journey.

- **28-Day Challenge:** Progress to a longer challenge for lasting change.

The principles of yoga have inspired millions over centuries, offering tools to overcome limitations and improve well-being. Chair yoga adapts this timeless wisdom, making it accessible to everyone and providing a pathway to relief and renewed movement. Join us on this journey of mindful movement, thousands of years in the making.

xiv

"The power of chair yoga

isn't in perfection—

it's in the practice."

— David Anthonie

Chapter 1

The Power of Chair Yoga

A Proven Practice Built on Ancient Principles

For centuries, people believed in yoga's ability to heal and restore—a belief now confirmed by modern science. Chair yoga carries this rich history forward, adapting its timeless principles into an easy and accessible practice. While once seen as alternative, these principles are now transforming lives everywhere.

By choosing this book, you've already taken a step toward hope, health, and healing—a path many have walked before you. Chair yoga offers a simple way to relieve pain, improve mobility, and enhance flexibility in just 10 minutes a day.

Mindful movement bridges ancient wisdom with modern needs, bringing yoga's benefits to everyone. With chair yoga, a life free from aches and pains is within reach—all from the comfort of a chair.

And the benefits don't stop at pain relief. Improved flexibility and mobility can bring with them new energy and reimagined possibilities. Chair yoga helps you rediscover the freedom to move with comfort and confidence—no experience required. This is your journey, and it starts here.

The Truth Behind Stiffness

Flexibility is about how far your muscles and joints can safely stretch and bend. Everybody's range of motion is different, and that's perfectly normal. Mobility refers to how easily and freely you can move your body. Just like flexibility, mobility can vary from person to person. They work together to help you move easily and comfortably, improving your quality of life.

Both flexibility and mobility are essential to staying independent and active as we age, and they play a crucial role in relieving aches and pains. When your muscles are tense, and your joints are tight, it can lead to stiffness and limit your ability to move freely. But with improved flexibility and mobility, you can reduce pain, increase your range of motion, and enjoy a more active lifestyle. It all begins by rediscovering your body's potential through chair yoga.

Familiar Poses with a Twist

If you've practiced yoga before, you might recognize some poses—but with a few twists. And that's okay! Chair yoga adapts poses to fit different needs and abilities. Our approach makes chair yoga simple and easy to follow, perfect for everyone.

Each routine is designed to be senior-friendly, with clear illustrations and simple instructions. For those who want to go deeper, our comprehensive Pose Library in Chapter 2 offers expanded guidance, modifications, and detailed illustrations to enhance your practice. These resources work together to help you get the most out of your chair yoga experience.

Fitness Made Simple

Have you tried fitness programs that left you feeling overwhelmed or discouraged—like they were made for someone else? We have, too. Many programs rely on complex routines and rigid challenges that can be hard to follow, especially for beginners or those dealing with aches, pains, or limited mobility. That's why we've designed a better way to experience the benefits of chair yoga—one that's gentle, effective, and adaptable to your needs.

This book offers a simple "less is more" approach to chair yoga that promises results that last. Instead of overwhelming you with too many poses and unrealistic challenges, we've carefully curated your plans with just the right balance. This allows you to make progress faster through repetition and achievable milestones, helping you build muscle memory, gain confidence, and enjoy the benefits of chair yoga without any unnecessary complications.

We keep everything simple with clear instructions in everyday language—no jargon or technical terms. Every exercise is accessible to everyone. Everything you need to start your chair yoga journey is right here in this book, with no hidden extras to download. Here's some of what you can expect:

- **Clear Benefits:** Each pose includes specific benefits to help you get the most out of your practice.
- **Simple Instructions:** We use everyday language and avoid technical terms, making it easy for everyone to follow along.
- **Clear Visuals:** Each pose includes large, easy-to-follow illustrations.
- **Modifications for Everybody:** Variations and modifications for each pose promote a safe and comfortable practice.

- **Short, Manageable Routines:** Our 10-minute routines fit seamlessly into your day, making it easy to experience the benefits of chair yoga.

- **Flexible Schedules:** Forget strict timelines and demanding expectations—this is your journey, at your own pace.

- **Gentle and Enjoyable:** We prioritize your well-being, encouraging you to listen to your body and modify poses as needed.

- **No Pressure and No Gimmicks:** Everything you need is right here in this book—no hidden extras to download.

- **Accessible and Convenient:** There's no need to get up and down from the floor, making it safe and accessible for those with limited mobility. All you need is a safe chair and comfortable clothing.

- **Practice Anywhere at Anytime:** Chair yoga can be done at home, in a park, at the gym, or even on your porch—anywhere you feel safe and comfortable with a sturdy chair.

- **Social or Solo:** Enjoy chair yoga on your own or connect with friends and family for a shared experience.

Chair yoga isn't about complexity or perfection—it's about consistent, gentle movements that help you reconnect with your body and uncover your hidden potential. With every milestone, you'll grow stronger, build confidence, and move closer to lasting change—one day at a time.

With all these benefits in mind, you might be wondering how to get started. In the next section, we'll guide you step by step, making it easy to follow each routine and build your practice at a pace that works for you.

Making This Book Work for You

This is your step-by-step guide to making chair yoga a meaningful part of your life. Follow along at a pace that feels right for you, and let your practice become both personal and powerful. Here are a few tips to help you get started and make the most of every page:

- **Begin with the Foundations:** Start from the beginning of the book to discover the transformative potential of chair yoga and its rich history.

- **Learn How Your Practice Will Grow:** Chapter 2 outlines the simple principles that form the foundation of your practice.

- **Familiarize Yourself with the Poses:** Explore The Pose Library in Chapter 2 with a comprehensive guide to each pose.

- **Understand the Phases of Your Journey:** Chapter 2 explains the practice and phases, showing you how to create lasting change.

- **Focus on Each Day's Routine:** Chapters 3 through 7 provide detailed instructions for daily routines, each targeting a specific area of the body.

- **Celebrate Your Milestones:** Chapter 8 recognizes your accomplishments and guides you toward transitioning chair yoga into a sustainable lifestyle practice.

- **Enjoy Each Step of the Journey:** This practice is about more than mindful movement—it's about connecting with your body, relieving pain, and finding balance.

This book is your guide, but the journey is yours to shape. Trust yourself, take your time, and find strength in simplicity. Above all, prioritize your safety and well-being. In the next section, you'll find essential tips to help you practice chair yoga safely and confidently.

A Safe Path to Mindful Movement

Your safety is the top priority. Throughout this book, you'll find modifications for each pose to help you practice safely and comfortably. These suggestions are meant to guide you as you explore and experiment. Find what works best for your body, and choose modifications that feel right for you. Here are some additional tips to help you create a safe and enjoyable practice:

- **Choose the Right Chair:** Use a sturdy chair without wheels, ensuring your feet can rest flat on the floor.

- **Consult Your Doctor:** If you have any health concerns, check with your doctor before starting any new exercise program.

- **Listen to Your Body:** Pay attention to how your body feels. If something causes discomfort, pause, rest, and make adjustments as needed.

- **Wear Comfortable Clothing:** Choose loose-fitting, comfortable clothing so you can move freely.

- **Create a Safe Space:** Practice in a clear, clutter-free area with enough room for movement.

- **Footwear:** Practice chair yoga barefoot or with comfortable, non-slip shoes—whichever feels safest and most comfortable.

- **Hydration:** Stay hydrated by drinking water before, during, and after your practice.

- **Use Modifications:** Adapt any pose to suit your comfort and needs.

- **Progress Gradually:** Start slowly then gradually increase the intensity as your strength and flexibility improve.

Everything starts with safety, but don't forget about the magic you can find in movement. Yes, the magic of movement. Remember those first clumsy moments of learning something new—like riding a bike or dancing? Every movement felt awkward and stiff, carefully calculated, as if your brain and body weren't quite in sync. There was no rhythm, just effort and uncertainty. No magic yet.

Then, something changed. Gradually, the movements began to flow, and it felt fluid and natural. For a brief, beautiful moment, everything clicked. You felt it—that indescribable sense of freedom, that perfect alignment of body and mind. The magic! It felt like anything was possible—and maybe it still is.

The Magic of Mindful Movement

Imagine still believing that anything is possible—that your childlike wonder is just waiting to be rediscovered. By approaching chair yoga with an open mind and letting go of limiting beliefs, you can unlock your hidden potential. You might even reconnect with who you used to be—the things you could do, the places you could go. Freedom. Movement could be the beginning of believing in possibilities again.

When you approach each pose with genuine curiosity and an open mind, the movements can guide you toward that same sense of freedom you once felt. This journey is about rediscovering yourself and realizing that the person you've been longing to be has been waiting for you all along. And all you have to do to find yourself again is believe.

It's not impossible. You've done it before—not by standing still, not by doing nothing. You changed your life by taking action. Maybe it started in your mind, and then your body followed—or maybe your body moved first, and your mind raced to catch up. Either way, you did something, and your world changed. What if there really is magic in movement, and chair yoga is the mindful movement that sparks the beginning of something amazing? Let's explore it together.

*"Mindful movement
is the magic
that reminds your body
it's never too late for miracles."*

— David Anthonie

Chapter 2

The Plan & The Poses

A Practice-Proven Path

Welcome to the heart of your chair yoga transformation! In this chapter, you'll discover a simple, effective plan to guide you on your journey toward greater flexibility, mobility, and relief from aches and pains. Before diving into each pose, let's outline your path to health and wellness—one built on centuries of yoga principles and inspired by millions of success stories.

The Power of Simplicity

There are hundreds of chair yoga poses and just as many variations and adaptations—but you don't need all of them at once. We've carefully selected the essential movements that focus on relieving aches and pains, improving mobility, and enhancing flexibility. By simplifying something complex, we've made it easier for you to focus on what matters. Practicing the right poses consistently will help you achieve faster, long-lasting results.

A Step-by-Step Plan

Your journey unfolds over four distinct phases, each building on the last to help you develop greater strength, mobility, and flexibility in a holistic way. This structured approach deepens your understanding, improves mind-muscle memory, and delivers consistent results. Here's a quick look at what's ahead:

- **The 7-Day Challenge:** Kickstart your journey with daily routines that build confidence and consistency, each targeting different areas.

- **The 14-Day Challenge:** Deepen your practice by repeating the routines from the first week, exploring new layers of each pose, and gradually expanding your range of motion.

- **The 21-Day Challenge:** Refine your understanding of the poses by increasing the focus and precision of your movements while building strength and stamina.

- **The 28-Day Challenge:** Build on your progress with purpose, making chair yoga a natural part of your day. This phase focuses on deepening your connection to the practice while continuing to improve mobility, flexibility, and the freedom to move comfortably.

Each phase builds on the last, both gradually and holistically. The poses flow seamlessly, creating a balanced and effective practice that supports your progress every step of the way. By the end of the 28-Day Challenge, chair yoga will feel like a natural part of your life—effortless and empowering, like second nature. Now, let's take a closer look at how the poses and routines work together, balancing mindful movement with simplicity.

Powerful Poses

Each day within the plan offers a balanced routine featuring five powerful poses. These aren't just any poses—we've carefully selected the most effective ones to help you get the most out of your practice. While these routines are designed to be effective, it's important to personalize your practice. Go at a pace that feels right for you, listen to your body, and take breaks as needed. Over time, work toward completing the full routines.

The Daily Routines

Each day targets a specific area of your body, helping you improve mobility, increase flexibility, and release muscle tension and joint stiffness. Let's take a sneak peek at what's to come—you'll find full details and instructions in the upcoming chapters. For now, here's an overview of your daily routines:

- **Day 1 Routine:** Release Neck & Shoulder Tension

- **Day 2 Routine:** Relieve Stiff Arms & Hands

- **Day 3 Routine:** Rescue Tired Legs & Feet

- **Day 4 Routine:** Reduce Back & Spine Pain

- **Day 5 Routine:** Restore Balance & Breathe

- **Rest Days:** The plan is designed for 5 days of routines followed by 2 rest days, but feel free to adjust the schedule to suit your needs. Listen to your body and take additional rest whenever it feels right for you.

Remember, these are just previews. The full routines are detailed in the upcoming chapters. Before we dive in, let's explore why mastering a few essential poses is the foundation of your success.

The Strength of Simple Steps

When it comes to learning something new, less is often more. This program embraces that proven principle and combines it with another time-tested approach: small steps, repeated often, bring the best results. Instead of overwhelming you with countless poses, we focus on just a few, practiced regularly. This method helps you safely and effectively build strength, flexibility, and balance while reducing the risk of injury.

Learning mindful movements is like learning any skill—it takes time and repetition. Think of it like riding a bike. At first, it feels wobbly and uncertain. But with practice, the movements become habits, and soon they feel like second nature. That's the power of muscle memory. Chair yoga works the same way. By practicing a few select poses regularly, you'll build familiarity and awareness, allowing your body to move with greater comfort and confidence.

Making mindful movements feel fluid relies on muscle memory, which makes repetition essential. Just as your mind learns through practice, so does your body. By focusing on a smaller set of poses, you'll master the movements and experience the benefits sooner. Repetition helps your mind and body work together as a team, building trust in your abilities and confidence in your movements.

Remember, this plan follows the simple, time-tested philosophy of less is more. It's thoughtfully crafted to be both straightforward and impactful, helping you enjoy the benefits of chair yoga without unnecessary complications. By focusing on key movements and practicing them consistently, you'll unlock lasting benefits that feel natural—not forced—and transform how you move and feel every day.

Let's face it—some things in life are hard and complicated—but chair yoga doesn't have to be. This simple method works with your body's natural rhythm, encouraging progress that feels effortless and sustainable, helping you build healthy habits naturally.

How Healthy Habits Happen

Building healthy habits takes time, consistency, and the right approach. Sound familiar? That's exactly how your chair yoga plan works—start small, build gradually, and gain momentum week by week. By the end of your 28-day journey, chair yoga will feel natural, like a healthy habit that's become part of your daily routine. Here's how each phase helps you build that habit:

- **Start Small and Build Gradually:** Habits begin with manageable steps. Starting with the 7-Day Challenge keeps things short and simple, helping you take action without feeling overwhelmed.

- **Make It Enjoyable:** Habits stick when they're enjoyable. During the 14-Day Challenge, you'll repeat familiar poses, explore new layers, and find joy in movement—a key to lasting habits.

- **Prioritize Safety and Recovery:** Progress happens when you feel safe. During the 21-Day Challenge, refining your movements builds confidence and control while lowering the risk of injury. And recovery isn't just rest—it's an essential part of progress, actively supporting your growth and ensuring lasting success.

- **Build Habits That Lead to Results:** Transformation comes from consistency. In the 28-Day Challenge, chair yoga starts to feel less like something you do and more like part of who you are —naturally.

The phases in this book align with the principles of healthy habit-building, turning repetition into routine and routine into a healthy lifestyle. In the next section, we'll explore how chair yoga can grow from a simple habit into a lasting lifestyle.

From Practice to Progress

The 7-Day Challenge is more than just a starting point—it's the foundation for an intentional, step-by-step journey. Each phase builds on the last, progressively strengthening your body and deepening your practice. This structured approach is designed to help you achieve sustainable changes, transforming chair yoga into a natural, lifelong practice.

Through repetition, your practice strengthens both muscle memory and the mind-muscle connection. Over time, this connection enables your fine motor skills, major muscle groups, ligaments, and tendons to work together seamlessly, supporting both everyday movements and overall stability.

- **Fine Motor Skills:** Improve tasks like buttoning a shirt or picking up small objects, making daily activities easier.

- **Major Muscle Groups:** Build strength for essential movements like standing up from a chair or carrying groceries.

- **Flexible Ligaments and Tendons:** Reduce the risk of injury while improving comfort in movements like bending to tie your shoes.

As your body learns to work together, you'll experience greater balance and alignment, which reduces aches, stiffness, and discomfort. Chair yoga helps restore this balance, promoting long-term health and well-being through gentle, purposeful movements.

By following this phased approach, you'll progress at a natural pace, building strength, balance, and flexibility with confidence. Now, let's take a closer look at how each day's routine is structured to guide your progress and deliver meaningful results.

Focus at Your Fingertips

Enjoy a seamless practice with our user-friendly design. Each day's routine is presented in its own dedicated chapter, with all the details you need in one place—no need to go searching for poses, pictures, instructions, or tips. Everything is organized to be easy to find and follow.

With this approach, you'll spend more time enjoying your practice and less time flipping through pages. Each daily routine chapter includes:

- **Previews:** A quick overview of the day's routine.
- **Full Page Layouts:** Each pose is presented on its own page.
- **Pictures:** Clear, helpful images to guide your movements.
- **Instructions:** Simple, step-by-step directions for every pose.
- **Guides:** Tips on breathing, modifications, safety, and benefits.

The daily routines feature the same poses from The Pose Library, presented in a condensed format for easy reference. For more detailed instructions or a closer look at any pose, simply return to The Pose Library whenever you want.

Our layout helps you stay focused on each pose, making it easier to enjoy your practice and get the most out of every movement. With all the details at your fingertips, there's no page flipping back and forth to break your flow. Let's take a closer look at how the poses are presented in The Pose Library.

The Look of The Library

The Pose Library introduces the essential movements that form the foundation of your practice, with each pose presented across a two-page layout. Here's what the layout looks like:

- **The Left Page:** A large, clear image with simple, step-by-step instructions in everyday language to guide your movements.

- **The Right Page:** Practical tips on breathing, safety, and modifications, plus a list of key benefits specific to each pose.

This design provides all the guidance you need to build confidence, master the movements, and support your growth at every stage of your journey. Whether you're learning a pose for the first time or revisiting it for greater insight, you'll find everything you need to let your chair yoga practice evolve naturally.

The Power of The Pose Library

The Pose Library prepares your path. Studying the left-page images and instructions and right-page tips strengthens both your mind and body by building the mind-muscle connection. This is what will make the movements feel natural and intuitive.

As you study, visualizing yourself performing each movement reinforces these connections, building familiarity and trust even before you begin. This step helps the routines in the Daily Routine chapters flow effortlessly. The more you understand the poses now, the more meaningful and rewarding your practice will be later.

Now that you're familiar with how The Pose Library works, it's time to explore the poses. Take your time reviewing each one, let them sink in, and remember—this isn't about memorizing. It's about getting familiar and building the mind-muscle connections before you even begin the movements. Let's get started!

*"Lasting change comes from steady steps, not leaps.
In chair yoga, every movement—
simple and repeated—becomes a stepping stone
to lifelong strength, flexibility, and balance."*

— David Anthonie

NECK ROLLS

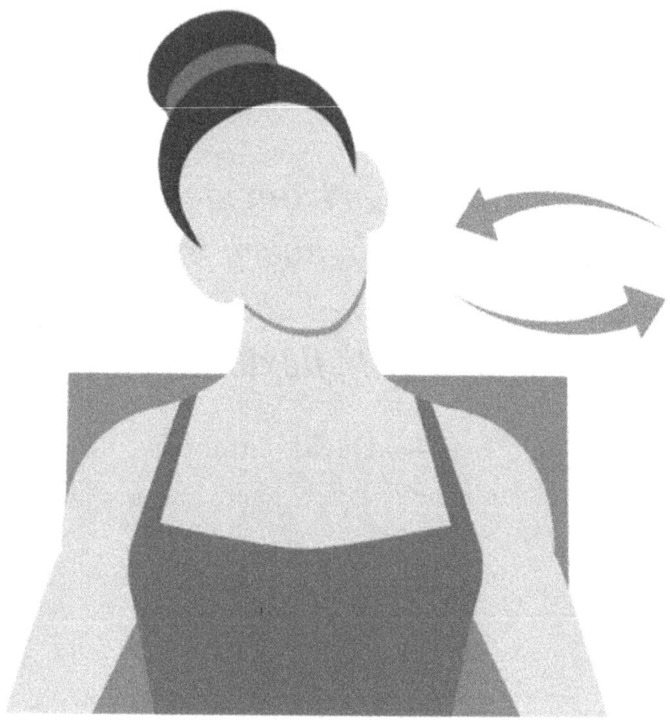

INSTRUCTIONS

1. Sit up straight with your feet flat on the floor.

2. Slowly tilt your right ear toward your right shoulder.

3. Gently roll your chin toward your chest.

4. Slowly tilt your left ear toward your left shoulder.

5. Gently roll your head to neutral.

6. Slowly switch directions.

7. Gently tilt your left ear toward your left shoulder.

8. Slowly roll your chin toward your chest.

9. Gently tilt your right ear toward your right shoulder.

10. Slowly roll your head to the center.

11. Continue alternating directions a few times or for as long as it feels good, then gently come to a stop.

NECK ROLLS

Breathing Guide

- Breathe naturally and comfortably throughout the exercise.

Modifications Guide

- Neck feeling stiff? Only tilt and roll your head as much as is comfortable.
- Dizziness or Vertigo? Avoid full neck rolls and focus on side-to-side head tilts instead.

Safety Guide

- Move slowly and smoothly. Avoid any sudden or jerky movements.
- Listen to your body. Stop if you feel any discomfort.
- Keep your shoulders loose. Don't lift or lock them.
- Don't stretch your neck too much. Only move it as much as is comfortable.

Benefits Guide

- Releases tension and stiffness in the neck and shoulders.
- Improves mobility and flexibility in the neck.
- Improves circulation in the head and neck.
- Improves mood and reduces stress.
- Improves posture and reduces joint pain.

SHOULDER SHRUGS

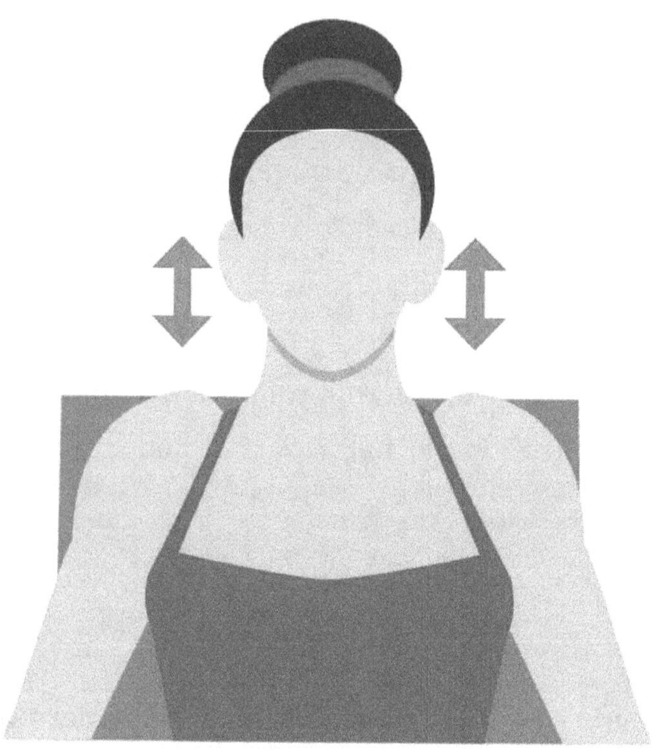

INSTRUCTIONS

1. Sit up straight with your feet flat on the floor.

2. Gently lift your shoulders toward your ears.

3. Briefly pause when your shoulders are at the top of the movement.

4. Slowly lower your shoulders down to their natural resting position.

5. Relax your shoulders at the bottom of the movement.

6. When you're ready, repeat the movement.

7. Repeat this movement a few times or for as long as it feels good, then gently come to a stop.

SHOULDER SHRUGS

Breathing Guide

- Inhale: As you lift your shoulders toward your ears.
- Exhale: As you lower your shoulders to a resting position.

* If the suggested breathing feels challenging or uncomfortable, breathe naturally and easily. As you become more familiar with the pose, you can gradually explore the suggested breathing pattern.

Modifications Guide

- Shoulders feeling stiff? Only move your shoulders as much as is comfortable.
- Feeling unsteady? Place both hands on your knees or thighs for balance.

Safety Guide

- Move slowly and smoothly. Avoid any sudden or jerky movements.
- Listen to your body. Stop if you feel any discomfort.
- Sit up straight and avoid rounding your shoulders forward.

Benefits Guide

- Improves mobility and flexibility in the neck and shoulders.
- Releases tension and stiffness in the neck and shoulders.
- Improves posture and reduces joint pain.
- Strengthens the shoulders and upper back.
- Improves mood and reduces stress.

CACTUS ARMS

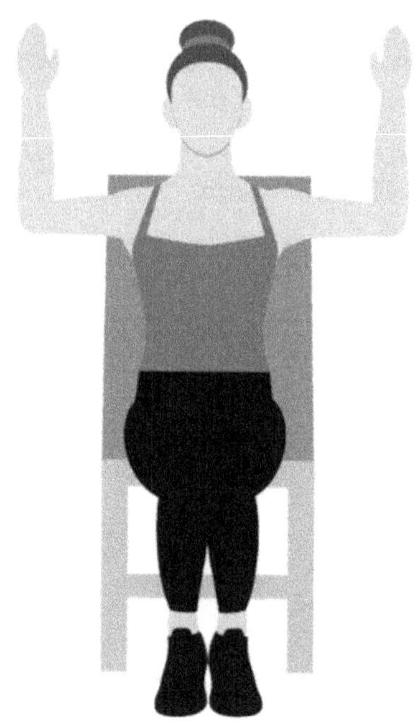 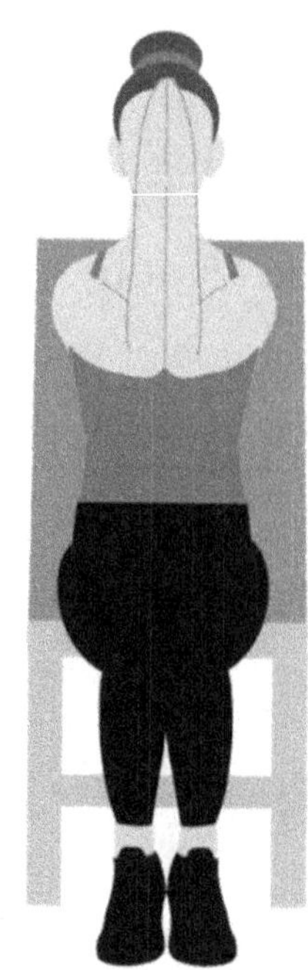

INSTRUCTIONS

1. Sit up straight with your feet flat on the floor.

2. Extend your arms to your sides with your palms facing down.

3. Bend your elbows to create an L-shape with your arms.

4. Gently rotate your forearms upward with your palms facing forward.

5. Slowly bring your forearms together until your palms touch.

6. Hold this position for a few breaths.

7. Slowly open your forearms to the sides until your palms face forward.

8. Repeat this movement a few times or for as long as it feels good, then gently come to a stop.

CACTUS ARMS

Breathing Guide

- Inhale: As you open your forearms to the sides.
- Exhale: As you bring your forearms together.

* If the suggested breathing feels challenging or uncomfortable, breathe naturally and easily. As you become more familiar with the pose, you can gradually explore the suggested breathing pattern.

Modifications Guide

- Shoulders feeling stiff? Only bring your forearms as close together as is comfortable.
- Wrists feeling stiff? Instead of pressing your palms together, gently touch your fingertips together.

Safety Guide

- Move slowly and smoothly. Avoid any sudden or jerky movements.
- Listen to your body. Stop if you feel any discomfort.
- Keep your shoulders loose. Don't lift or lock them.

Benefits Guide

- Improves mobility and flexibility in the shoulders and upper back.
- Strengthens the shoulders and upper back.
- Improves posture and reduces joint pain.
- Reduces tightness in the chest and helps improve breathing.

CAT COW POSE

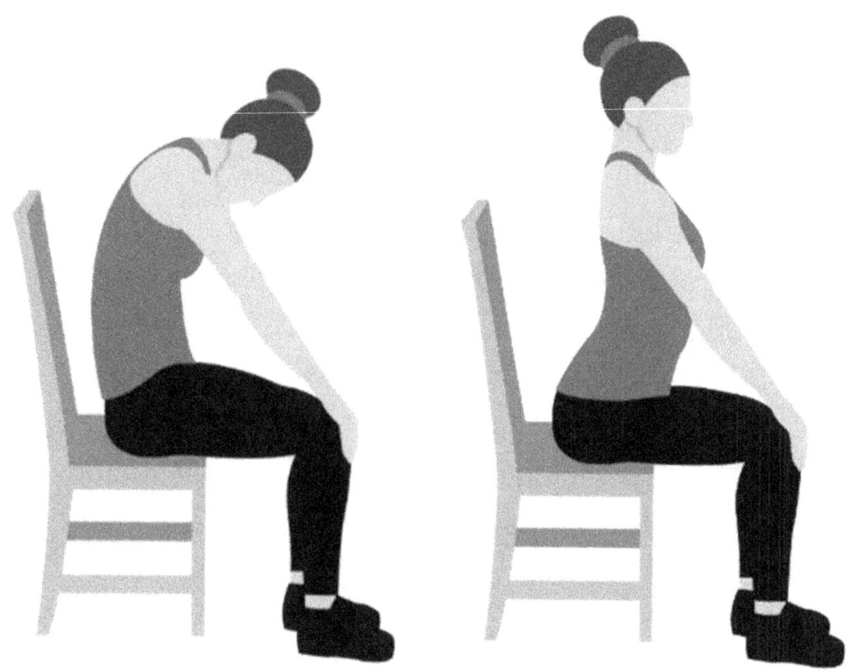

INSTRUCTIONS

1. Sit up straight with your feet flat on the floor.

2. Place both hands on your knees.

3. Slowly curl your back like a cat and drop your chin.

4. Hold this pose for a few breaths, then slowly switch directions.

5. Gently lift your chest and slowly dip your back like a cow.

6. Hold this pose for a few breaths, then gently sit up straight.

7. When you're ready, repeat the movement.

8. Continue alternating poses a few times or for as long as it feels good, then gently come to a stop.

CAT COW POSE

Breathing Guide

- Inhale: As you curl your back like a cat and drop your chin.
- Exhale: As you lift your chest and dip your lower back like a cow.

* If the suggested breathing feels challenging or uncomfortable, breathe naturally and easily. As you become more familiar with the pose, you can gradually explore the suggested breathing pattern.

Modifications Guide

- Back feeling stiff? Only arch and dip your back as much as is comfortable.
- Neck feeling stiff? Only move your head as much as is comfortable.

Safety Guide

- Move slowly and gently. No sudden or jerky movements.
- Listen to your body. Stop if you feel any discomfort.
- Keep your shoulders loose. Don't lift or lock them.

Benefits Guide

- Improves mobility and flexibility in your back and shoulders.
- Releases tension and stiffness in your back and shoulders.
- It may help stimulate digestion and soothe mild stomach discomfort.
- Improves mood and reduces stress.
- Improves posture and reduces joint pain.

SEATED TWIST

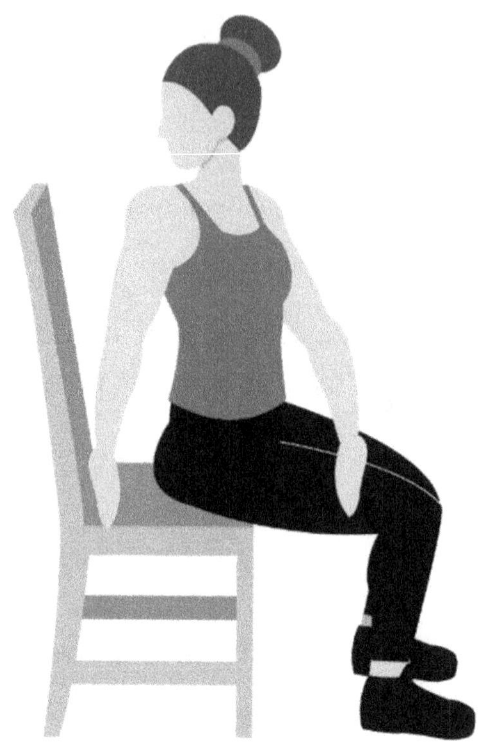

INSTRUCTIONS

1. Sit up straight with your feet flat on the floor.

2. Place your right hand behind you on the chair.

3. Place your left hand on the outside of your right thigh.

4. Gently twist to the right and look over your right shoulder.

5. Hold this pose for a few breaths, then slowly switch sides.

6. Place your left hand behind you on the chair.

7. Place your right hand on the outside of your left thigh.

8. Gently twist to the left and look over your left shoulder.

9. Continue alternating sides a few times or for as long as it feels good, then gently come to a stop.

SEATED TWIST

Breathing Guide

- Inhale: As you sit up straight and prepare to twist.
- Exhale: As you gently twist your body.

* If the suggested breathing feels challenging or uncomfortable, breathe naturally and easily. As you become more familiar with the pose, you can gradually explore the suggested breathing pattern.

Modifications Guide

- Back feeling stiff? Only twist your body as much as is comfortable.
- Neck feeling stiff? Only turn your head as much as is comfortable.
- Shoulder feeling stiff? Place both hands on your thighs while you twist.

Safety Guide

- Move slowly and gently. No sudden or jerky movements.
- Listen to your body. Stop if you feel any discomfort.
- Don't over-twist. The stretch should feel good, not uncomfortable.

Benefits Guide

- Improves mobility and flexibility in the back.
- It may help stimulate digestion and soothe mild stomach discomfort.
- Releases tension and stiffness in the back, shoulders, and chest.
- Improves mood and reduces stress.
- Improves posture and reduces joint pain.

WRIST CIRCLES

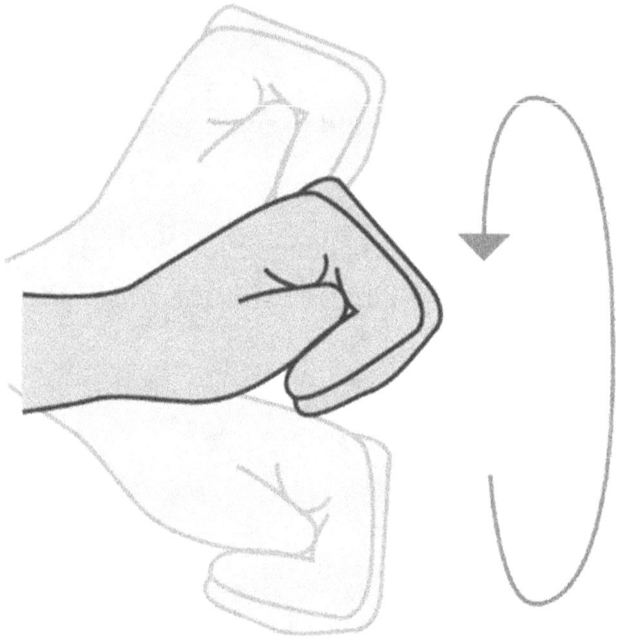

INSTRUCTIONS

1. Sit up straight with your feet flat on the floor.

2. Extend your arms to the front at chest level.

3. Slowly make soft fists with both of your hands.

4. Gently rotate your wrists in one direction, gradually making bigger circles.

5. Continue circling your wrists for a few breaths, then slowly change directions.

6. Gently rotate your wrists in the opposite direction, gradually making bigger circles.

7. Continue alternating directions a few times or for as long as it feels good, then gently come to a stop.

WRIST CIRCLES

Breathing Guide

- Breathe naturally and comfortably throughout the exercise.

Modifications Guide

- Wrists feeling stiff? Only rotate your wrists as much as is comfortable.
- Hands feeling stiff? Gently open and close your hands a few times before you begin.

Safety Guide

- Move slowly and gently. No sudden or jerky movements.
- Listen to your body. Stop if you feel any discomfort.
- Avoid locking your elbows. Keep them soft and slightly bent.

Benefits Guide

- Improves mobility and flexibility in the wrists.
- Releases tension and stiffness in the hands and wrists.
- Strengthens your wrists and forearms.
- Improves circulation in your wrists and hands.
- Improves mobility and flexibility in your wrists and hands.

WRIST SHAKES

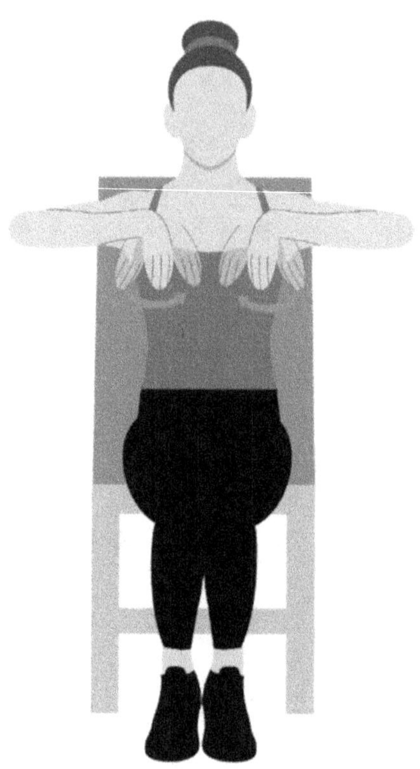

INSTRUCTIONS

1. Sit up straight with your feet flat on the floor.

2. Bend your elbows, then raise your forearms and hands to your chest.

3. Gently shake your hands and wrists from side to side.

4. Continue shaking for a few breaths, then rest your arms comfortably.

5. When you're ready, repeat the movement.

6. Bend your elbows, then raise your forearms and hands to your chest.

7. Gently adjust the shaking to a comfortable speed and intensity.

8. Repeat this movement a few times or for as long as it feels good, then gently come to a stop.

WRIST SHAKES

Breathing Guide

- Breathe naturally and comfortably throughout the exercise.

Modifications Guide

- Wrists feeling stiff? Only shake your wrists as much as is comfortable.
- Arms feeling stiff? Lower your arms down to your sides and shake your wrists there.

Safety Guide

- Begin with gentle shakes and gradually increase the intensity.
- Move slowly and gently. No sudden or jerky movements.
- Listen to your body. Stop if you feel any discomfort.

Benefits Guide

- Improves mobility and flexibility in your wrists and hands.
- Releases tension and stiffness in the hands and wrists.
- Improves circulation in your wrists and hands.

ARM CIRCLES

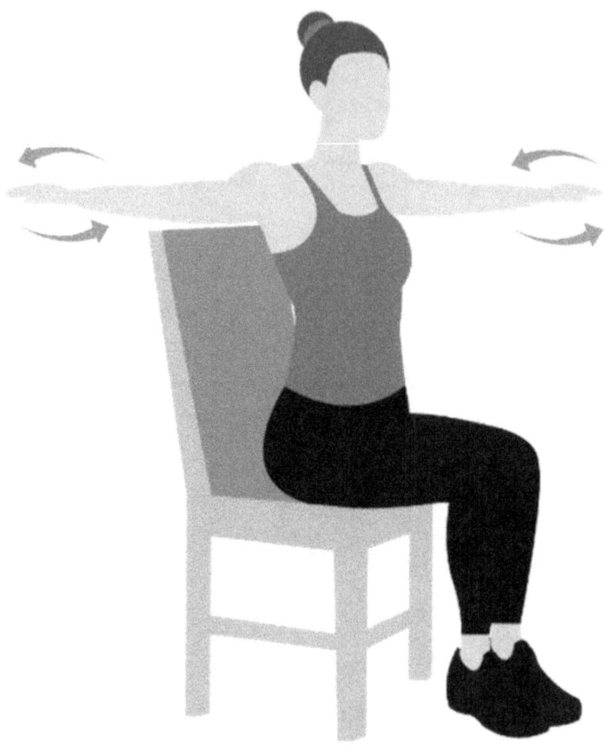

INSTRUCTIONS

1. Sit up straight with your feet flat on the floor.

2. Extend your arms to your sides with your palms facing down.

3. Slowly make small circles with your arms, moving them forward.

4. Gradually make the circles bigger as you feel comfortable.

5. Gently change directions.

6. Slowly make small circles with your arms, moving them backward.

7. Gradually make the circles bigger as you feel comfortable.

8. Continue alternating directions a few times or for as long as it feels good, then gently come to a stop.

ARM CIRCLES

Breathing Guide

- Inhale: As you circle your arms forward.
- Exhale: As you circle your arms backward.

* If the suggested breathing feels challenging or uncomfortable, breathe naturally and easily. As you become more familiar with the pose, you can gradually explore the suggested breathing pattern.

Modifications Guide

- Shoulders feeling stiff? Only move your arms as much as is comfortable.
- Arms feeling stiff? Lower your arms down to your sides and make arm circles there.
- Wrists feeling stiff? Make loose fists as you circle your arms.

Safety Guide

- Move slowly and gently. No sudden or jerky movements.
- Listen to your body. Stop if you feel any discomfort.
- Keep your shoulders loose. Don't lift or lock them.

Benefits Guide

- Improves mobility and flexibility in the shoulders.
- Releases tension and stiffness in the shoulders and upper back.
- Strengthens the shoulders and arms.
- Improves circulation in the shoulders and arms.

WRIST STRETCHES

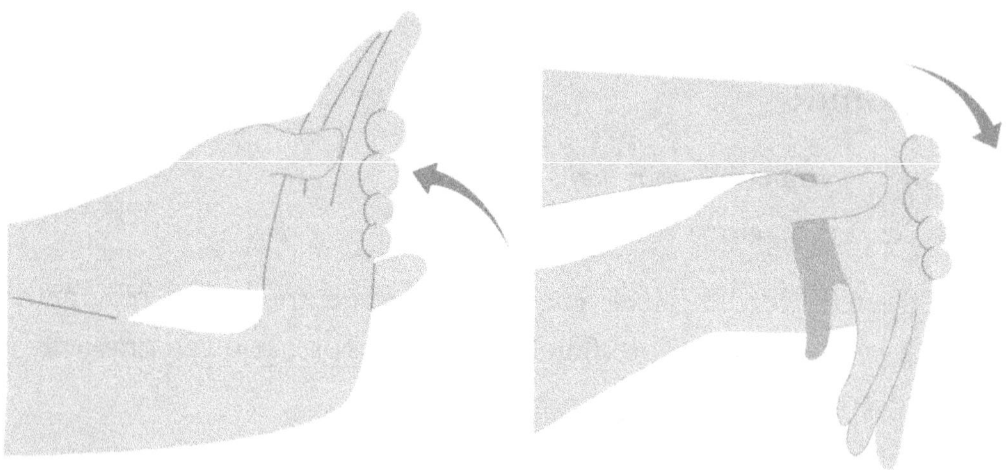

INSTRUCTIONS

1. Sit up straight with your feet flat on the floor.

2. Extend one arm to the front with your palm facing down.

3. Slowly extend your wrist backward with your fingers toward the sky.

4. Gently assist in bending your wrist backward with the other hand.

5. Hold this pose for a few breaths, then switch directions.

6. Gently flex your wrist forward with your fingers toward the floor.

7. Gently assist in bending your wrist forward with the other hand.

8. Slowly switch to the other arm and repeat.

9. Continue alternating directions and arms a few times or for as long as it feels good, then gently come to a stop.

WRIST STRETCHES

Breathing Guide

- Breathe naturally and comfortably throughout the exercise.

Modifications Guide

- Wrists feeling stiff? Only bend your wrist as much as is comfortable.
- Hands feeling stiff? Spread your fingers wide a few times before starting.

Safety Guide

- Move slowly and gently. No sudden or jerky movements.
- Listen to your body. Stop if you feel any discomfort.
- Keep your shoulders loose. Don't lift or lock them.

Benefits Guide

- Improves mobility and flexibility in your wrists and hands.
- Releases tension and stiffness in the hands and wrists.
- Improves circulation in your wrists and hands.

EAGLE ARMS

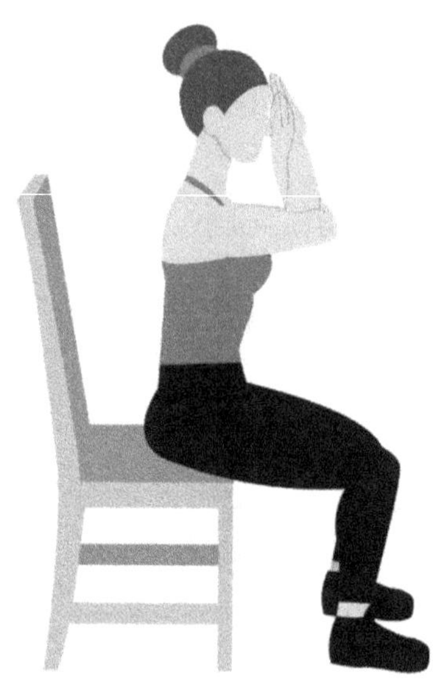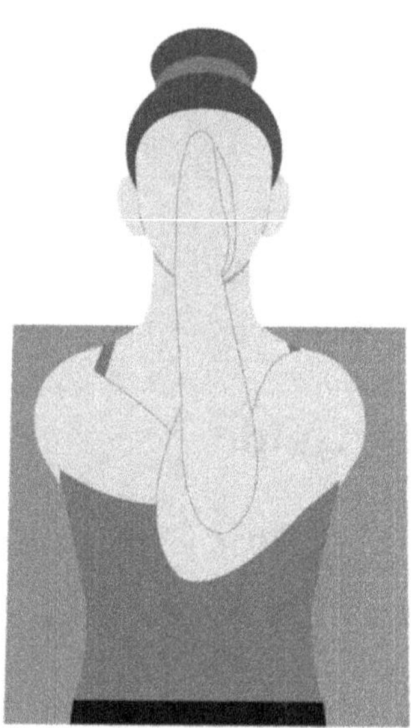

INSTRUCTIONS

1. Sit up straight with your feet flat on the floor.

2. Cross your left elbow over your right elbow.

3. Gently bend your elbows and crisscross your forearms.

4. Slowly lift your elbows and bring the backs of your hands together.

5. Hold this pose for a few breaths, then slowly switch sides.

6. Cross your right elbow over your left elbow.

7. Gently bend your elbows and crisscross your forearms.

8. Slowly lift your elbows and bring the backs of your hands together.

9. Hold this pose for a few breaths, then rest your arms comfortably.

10. When you're ready, repeat the movement.

11. Continue alternating arms a few times or for as long as it feels good, then gently come to a stop.

EAGLE ARMS

Breathing Guide

- Inhale: As you extend your arms to the front.
- Exhale: As you cross your arms and gently bend your elbows.

* If the suggested breathing feels challenging or uncomfortable, breathe naturally and easily. As you become more familiar with the pose, you can gradually explore the suggested breathing pattern.

Modifications Guide

- Shoulders feeling stiff? Give yourself a big hug instead, reaching your arms across your chest and holding the opposite shoulders.
- Can't cross your elbows? Cross your wrists instead, then press the backs of your hands together.

Safety Guide

- Move slowly and gently. No sudden or jerky movements.
- Listen to your body. Stop if you feel any discomfort.
- Keep your shoulders loose. Don't lift or lock them.
- Don't over-stretch. The stretch should feel good, not uncomfortable.

Benefits Guide

- Improves mobility and flexibility in the shoulders, upper back, and neck.
- Improves circulation in the shoulders, upper back, and neck.
- Releases tension and stiffness in the shoulders, upper back, and neck.
- Improves mental focus, concentration, and coordination.

ANKLE CIRCLES

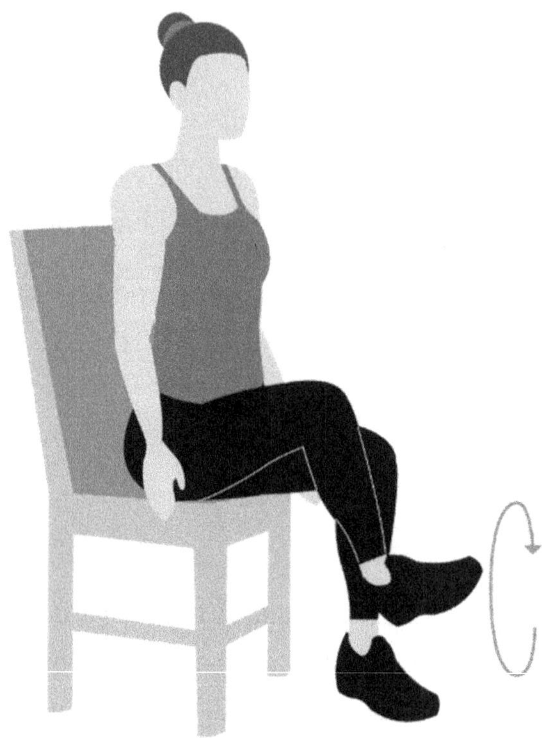

INSTRUCTIONS

1. Sit up straight with your feet flat on the floor.

2. Find a comfortable place to rest your hands.

3. Gently lift your right foot off the floor.

4. Slowly make circles with that ankle, gradually making bigger circles.

5. Gently change directions, gradually making bigger circles.

6. Slowly lower your right foot and switch to the other ankle.

7. Gently lift your left foot off the floor.

9. Slowly make circles with that ankle, gradually making bigger circles.

8. Gently change directions, gradually making bigger circles.

9. Slowly lower your left foot, resting both feet flat on the floor.

10. Continue alternating directions and sides a few times or for as long as it feels good, then gently come to a stop.

ANKLE CIRCLES

Breathing Guide

- Breathe naturally and comfortably throughout the exercise.

Modifications Guide

- Feet feeling stiff? Only make the circles as big as is comfortable.
- Feeling unsteady? Place both hands on your knees or thighs for balance.
- Foot feeling heavy? Slide your foot forward, then back, or side to side on the floor instead of making circles.

Safety Guide

- Move slowly and smoothly. Avoid any sudden or jerky movements.
- Listen to your body. Stop if you feel any discomfort.
- Sit up straight and avoid rounding your shoulders forward.

Benefits Guide

- Improves mobility and flexibility in the ankles and feet.
- Releases tension and stiffness in the ankles and feet.
- Reduces the risk of slips and falls by strengthening the ankles and feet.
- Improves circulation in the feet and ankles, which can help with swelling.

TOE RAISES

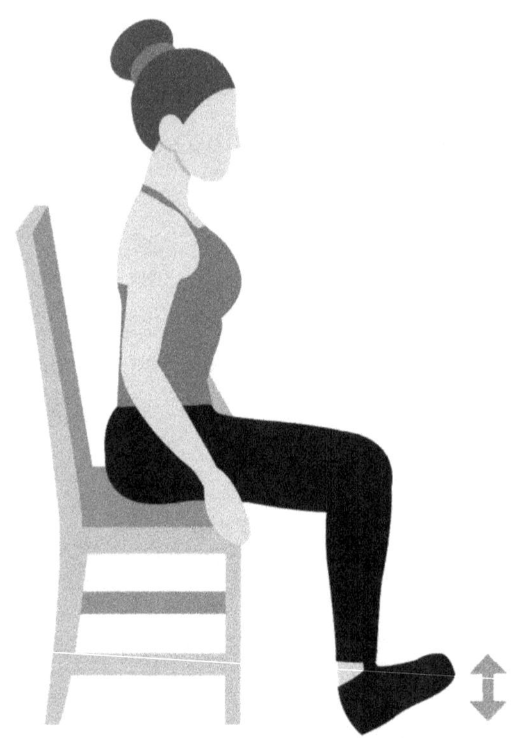

INSTRUCTIONS

1. Sit up straight with your feet flat on the floor.

2. Find a comfortable place to rest your hands.

3. Lift your toes, keeping your heels on the floor.

4. Hold this pose for a few breaths.

5. Slowly lower your toes until both feet are flat on the floor.

6. When you're ready, repeat the movement.

7. Repeat this movement a few times or for as long as it feels good, then gently come to a stop.

TOE RAISES

Breathing Guide

- Inhale: As you lift your toes.
- Exhale: As you lower your toes.

* If the suggested breathing feels challenging or uncomfortable, breathe naturally and easily. As you become more familiar with the pose, you can gradually explore the suggested breathing pattern.

Modifications Guide

- Ankles feeling stiff? Only lift your toes as much as is comfortable.
- Feeling unsteady? Place both hands on your knees or thighs for balance.

Safety Guide

- Move slowly and smoothly. Avoid any sudden or jerky movements.
- Listen to your body. Stop if you feel any discomfort.
- Keep your back straight and avoid rounding your shoulders forward.
- Keep your ankles steady. Avoid rolling them inward or outward.

Benefits Guide

- Improves mobility and flexibility in the ankles and feet.
- Releases tension and stiffness in the ankles and feet.
- Improves circulation in your feet and ankles, which can help with swelling.
- Reduces the risk of slips and falls by strengthening the ankles and feet.

FORWARD BEND

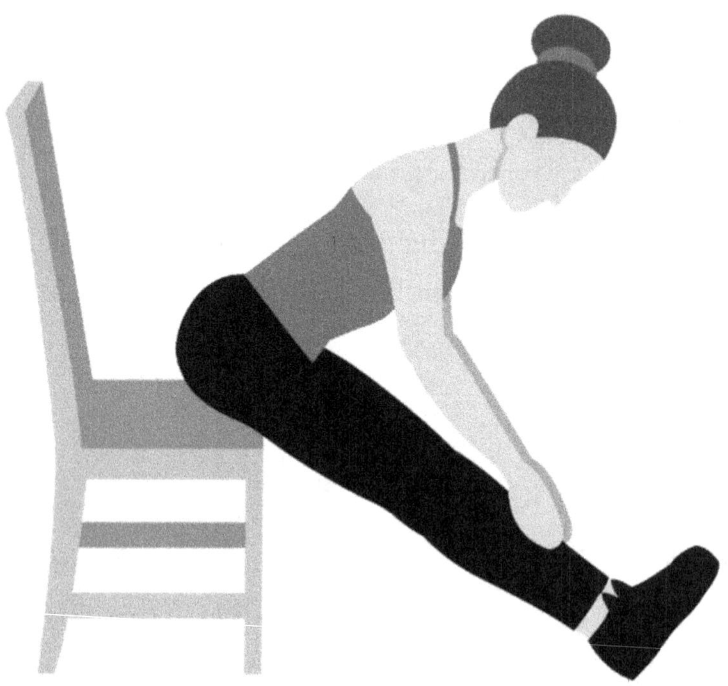

INSTRUCTIONS

1. Sit up straight near the front of the chair.

2. Extend your legs with your heels on the floor.

3. Slowly bend forward from your hips, keeping your back straight.

4. Gently reach for your ankles with your hands, extending your arms.

5. Hold this pose for a few breaths, then slowly sit up straight.

6. Relax your arms, legs, and feet by gently wiggling them.

7. When you're ready, repeat the movement.

8. Repeat this movement a few times or for as long as it feels good, then gently come to a stop.

FORWARD BEND

Breathing Guide

- Inhale: As you sit up straight and prepare to bend forward.
- Exhale: As you bend forward.

* If the suggested breathing feels challenging or uncomfortable, breathe naturally and easily. As you become more familiar with the pose, you can gradually explore the suggested breathing pattern.

Modifications Guide

- Legs feeling stiff? Bend your knees slightly for comfort.
- Back feeling stiff? Only bend forward as far as is comfortable.

Safety Guide

- Move slowly and smoothly. Avoid any sudden or jerky movements.
- Listen to your body. Stop if you feel any discomfort.
- Keep your back straight and avoid rounding your shoulders forward.

Benefits Guide

- Improves mobility and flexibility in the legs and back.
- It may help stimulate digestion and soothe mild stomach discomfort.
- Improves circulation in the lower body, which may help reduce swelling in the legs and feet.
- •Improves posture and reduces joint pain.
- Releases tension and stiffness in the lower back, shoulders, and hips.

QUAD STRETCH

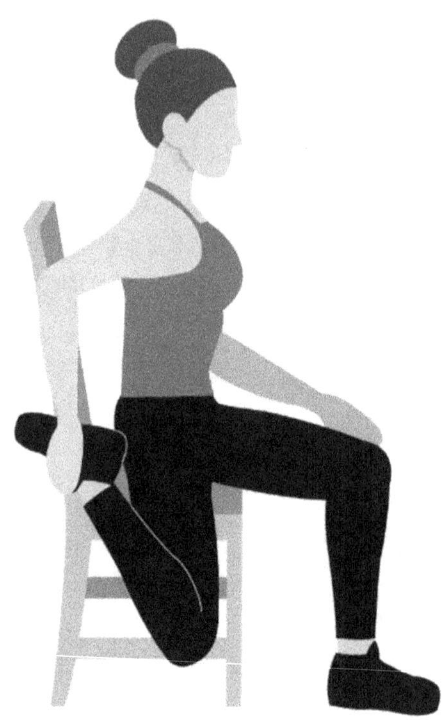

INSTRUCTIONS

1. Sit up straight with your feet flat on the floor.

2. Place your left hand on your left knee.

3. Slowly bend your right knee, bringing that foot behind you.

4. Gently pull your right foot toward your right hip.

5. Hold this pose for a few breaths, then slowly sit up straight.

6. Slowly switch sides.

7. Place your right hand on your right knee.

8. Slowly bend your left knee, bringing that foot behind you.

9. Gently pull your left foot toward your left hip.

10. Continue alternating sides a few times or for as long as it feels good, then gently come to a stop.

QUAD STRETCH

Breathing Guide

- Inhale: As you sit up straight and prepare to bend your knee.
- Exhale: As you pull your foot toward your hip.

* If the suggested breathing feels challenging or uncomfortable, breathe naturally and easily. As you become more familiar with the pose, you can gradually explore the suggested breathing pattern.

Modifications Guide

- Knee feeling stiff? Only bend your knee as much as is comfortable.
- Feeling unsteady? Hold onto the side of your chair with your free hand.

Safety Guide

- Move slowly and smoothly. Avoid any sudden or jerky movements.
- Listen to your body. Stop if you feel any discomfort.
- Don't pull too hard. The stretch should feel good, not painful.
- Keep your back straight and avoid leaning forward.

Benefits Guide

- Improves mobility and flexibility in the knees and legs.
- Releases tension and stiffness in the knees and legs
- Improves circulation in the legs.
- Improves posture and reduces joint pain.

HEEL RAISES

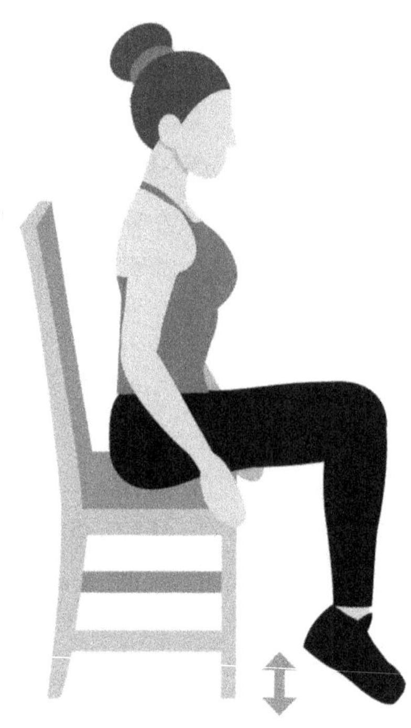

INSTRUCTIONS

1. Sit up straight with your feet flat on the floor.

2. Find a comfortable place to rest your hands.

3. Lift your heels, keeping your toes on the floor.

4. Hold this pose for a few breaths.

5. Slowly lower your heels until both feet are flat on the floor.

6. When you're ready, repeat the movement.

7. Repeat this movement a few times or for as long as it feels good, then gently come to a stop.

HEEL RAISES

Breathing Guide

- Inhale: As you lift your heels.
- Exhale: As you lower your heels.

* If the suggested breathing feels challenging or uncomfortable, breathe naturally and easily. As you become more familiar with the pose, you can gradually explore the suggested breathing pattern.

Modifications Guide

- Feet feeling stiff? Only lift your heels as much as is comfortable.
- Ankles feeling stiff? Lift one heel at a time, alternating between sides.
- Feeling unsteady? Place both hands on your knees or thighs for balance.

Safety Guide

- Move slowly and smoothly. Avoid any sudden or jerky movements.
- Listen to your body. Stop if you feel any discomfort.
- Sit up tall. Keep your back straight and avoid leaning.

Benefits Guide

- Reduces the risk of slips and falls by strengthening the calves, feet, and ankles.
- Improves circulation in the feet, ankles, and calves, which can help with swelling.
- Improves mobility and flexibility in the feet, ankles, and calves.
- Releases tension and stiffness in the feet, ankles, and calves.

FORWARD FOLD

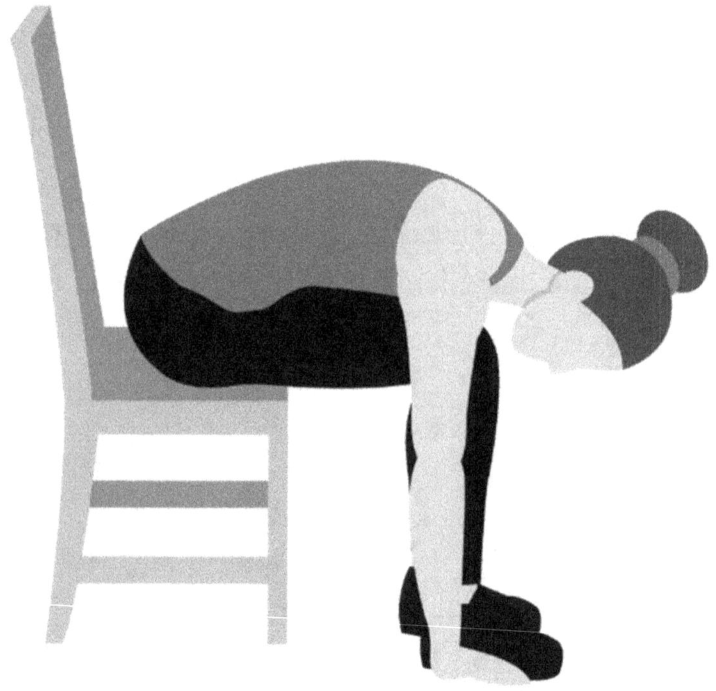

INSTRUCTIONS

1. Sit up straight near the front of your chair with your feet flat on the floor.

2. Slowly bend forward from your hips, bringing your chest toward your legs.

3. Gently reach your hands toward the floor, extending your arms.

4. Hold this pose for a few breaths, then slowly sit up straight.

5. When you're ready, repeat the movement.

6. Repeat this movement a few times or for as long as it feels good, then gently come to a stop.

FORWARD FOLD

Breathing Guide

- Inhale: As you sit up straight and prepare to fold forward.
- Exhale: As you fold forward.

* If the suggested breathing feels challenging or uncomfortable, breathe naturally and easily. As you become more familiar with the pose, you can gradually explore the suggested breathing pattern.

Modifications Guide

- Back feeling stiff? Only fold forward as much as is comfortable.
- Feeling unsteady? Place your hands on your knees or thighs for balance.

Safety Guide

- Move slowly and smoothly. Avoid any sudden or jerky movements.
- Listen to your body. Stop if you feel any discomfort.
- Keep your core engaged and avoid rounding your shoulders forward.

Benefits Guide

- Improves posture and reduces joint pain.
- It may help stimulate digestion and soothe mild stomach discomfort.
- Releases tension and stiffness in the lower back, shoulders, and hips.
- Improves mood and reduces stress.

COBRA POSE

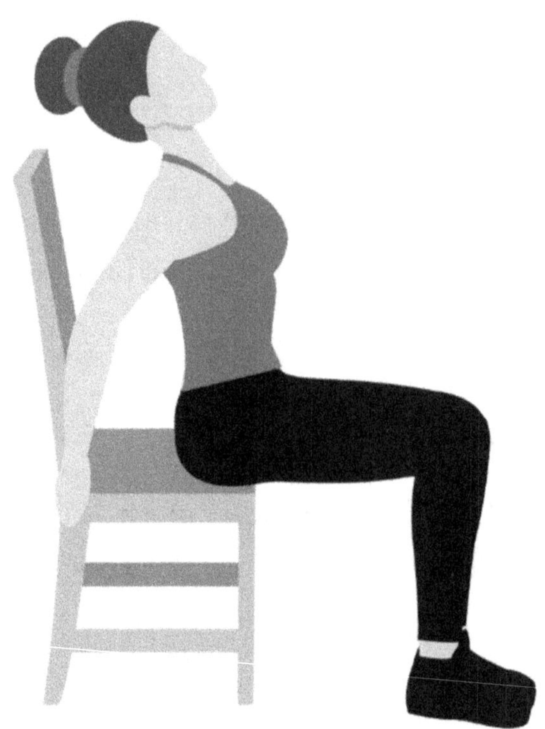

INSTRUCTIONS

1. Sit up straight near the front of your chair with your feet flat on the floor.

2. Gently place your hands behind you on the chair.

3. Slowly arch your upper back and lift your chest.

4. Gently tilt your chin upward.

5. Hold this pose for a few breaths.

6. Slowly sit up straight and lower your chest and chin.

7. When you're ready, repeat the movement.

8. Repeat this movement a few times or for as long as it feels good, then gently come to a stop.

COBRA POSE

Breathing Guide

- Inhale: As you arch your back and lift your chest and chin.
- Exhale: As you sit up straight and lower your chest and chin.

* If the suggested breathing feels challenging or uncomfortable, breathe naturally and easily. As you become more familiar with the pose, you can gradually explore the suggested breathing pattern.

Modifications Guide

- Back feeling stiff? Only arch your back as much as is comfortable.
- Neck feeling stiff? Only tilt your chin as much as is comfortable.

Safety Guide

- Move slowly and smoothly. Avoid any sudden or jerky movements.
- Listen to your body. Stop if you feel any discomfort.
- Keep your shoulders loose. Don't lift or lock them.

Benefits Guide

- Improves mobility and flexibility in the back, chest, and neck.
- Enhances breathing by stretching the chest, making it easier to breathe.
- Strengthens the back muscles, which can improve posture.
- Improves mood and reduces stress.
- Releases tension and stiffness in the upper back, chest, shoulders, and neck.

WIDE-LEGGED TWIST

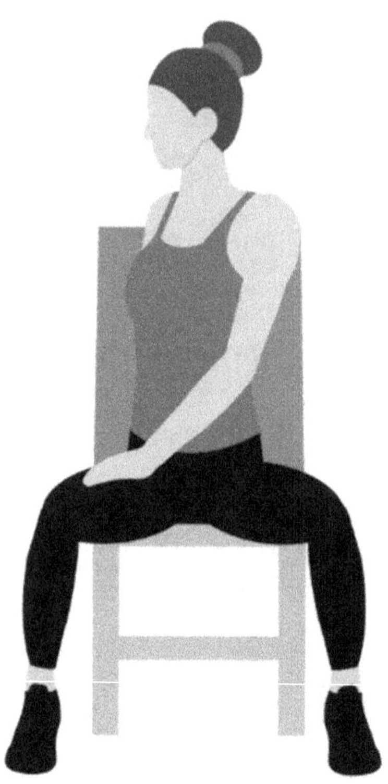

INSTRUCTIONS

1. Sit up straight near the front of your chair with your feet flat on the floor.

2. Place your right hand behind you on the chair and your left hand on your right thigh.

3. Gently turn your body to the right and look over your right shoulder.

4. Hold this pose for a few breaths and then slowly switch sides.

5. Place your left hand behind you on the chair and your right hand on your left thigh.

6. Gently turn your body to the left and look over your left shoulder.

7. Continue alternating sides a few times or for as long as it feels good, then gently come to a stop.

WIDE-LEGGED TWIST

Breathing Guide

- Inhale: As you sit up straight and prepare to turn your body.
- Exhale: As you turn your body.

* If the suggested breathing feels challenging or uncomfortable, breathe naturally and easily. As you become more familiar with the pose, you can gradually explore the suggested breathing pattern.

Modifications Guide

- Back feeling stiff? Only turn as much as is comfortable.
- Knees feeling stiff? Bring your feet closer together.
- Neck feeling stiff? Only turn your head as much as is comfortable.

Safety Guide

- Move slowly and smoothly. Avoid any sudden or jerky movements.
- Listen to your body. Stop if you feel any discomfort.
- Don't over-twist. Only turn as much as is comfortable.

Benefits Guide

- Improves mobility and flexibility in the back, shoulders, sides, and hips.
- Releases tension and stiffness in the back, shoulders, sides, and hips.
- It may help stimulate digestion and soothe mild stomach discomfort.
- Improves posture and reduces joint pain.
- Improves mood and reduces stress.

SIDE STRETCHES

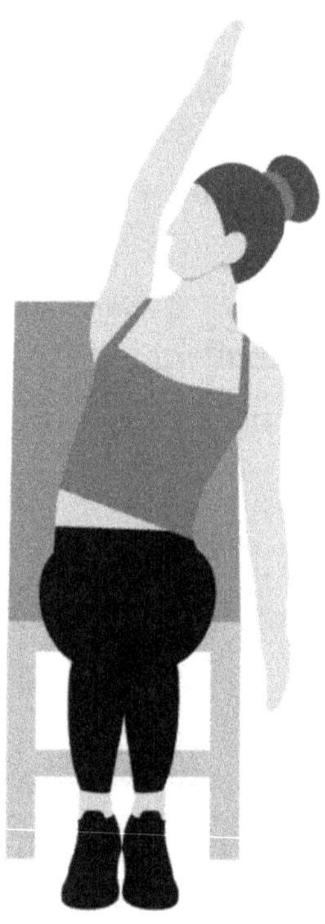

INSTRUCTIONS

1. Sit up straight with your feet flat on the floor.

2. Slowly raise your right arm toward the sky with your palm facing inward.

3. Gently reach your left arm down, bending your body to the left.

4. Hold this pose for a few breaths, then slowly switch sides.

5. Slowly raise your left arm toward the sky with your palm facing inward.

6. Gently reach your right arm down, bending your body to the right.

7. Continue alternating sides a few times or for as long as it feels good, then gently come to a stop.

SIDE STRETCHES

Breathing Guide

- Inhale: As you reach your raised arm toward the sky.
- Exhale: As you bend your body to the side.

* If the suggested breathing feels challenging or uncomfortable, breathe naturally and easily. As you become more familiar with the pose, you can gradually explore the suggested breathing pattern.

Modifications Guide

- Sides feeling stiff? Only bend your body as much as is comfortable.
- Shoulder feeling stiff? Rest your raised hand on the top of your head.
- Can't reach down? Rest your lower hand comfortably on your leg.

Safety Guide

- Move slowly and smoothly. Avoid any sudden or jerky movements.
- Listen to your body. Stop if you feel any discomfort.
- Don't overstretch. Only bend as much as is comfortable.

Benefits Guide

- Improves mobility and flexibility in the back, sides, and shoulders.
- Enhances breathing by stretching the chest, making it easier to breathe.
- Improves posture and reduces joint pain.
- Releases tension and stiffness in the sides, shoulders, upper back, and hips.
- Improves mood and reduces stress.

EXTENDED SIDE ANGLE POSE

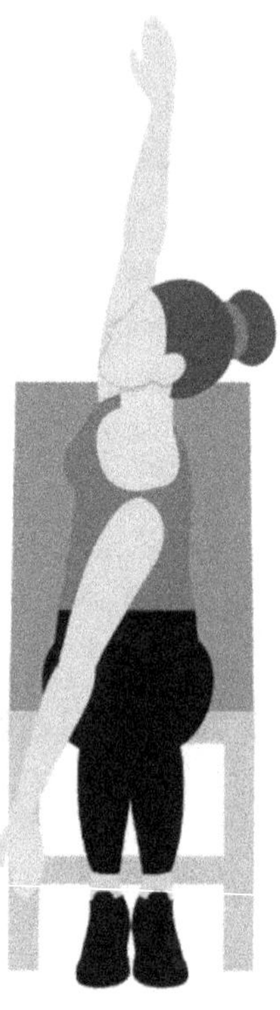

INSTRUCTIONS

1. Sit up straight near the front of the chair with your feet flat on the floor.

2. Slowly raise your right arm toward the sky, turning gently to the right.

3. Slowly reach your left hand toward the outside of your right foot.

4. Gently turn your body to the right as much as is comfortable.

5. Hold this pose for a few breaths, then slowly switch sides.

6. Slowly raise your left arm toward the sky, turning gently to the left.

7. Slowly reach your right hand down toward the outside of your left foot.

8. Gently turn your body to the left as much as is comfortable.

9. Continue alternating sides a few times or for as long as it feels good, then gently come to a stop.

EXTENDED SIDE ANGLE POSE

Breathing Guide

- Inhale: As you reach your raised arm toward the sky.
- Exhale: As you reach your lower arm toward your foot.

* If the suggested breathing feels challenging or uncomfortable, breathe naturally and easily. As you become more familiar with the pose, you can gradually explore the suggested breathing pattern.

Modifications Guide

- Back feeling stiff? Only turn your body as much as is comfortable.
- Shoulder feeling stiff? Rest your raised hand on the top of your head.
- Feeling unsteady? Rest your lower hand comfortably on your leg.

Safety Guide

- Move slowly and smoothly. Avoid any sudden or jerky movements.
- Listen to your body. Stop if you feel any discomfort.
- Don't overtwist. Only turn your body as much as is comfortable.

Benefits Guide

- Improves mobility and flexibility in the sides, shoulders, back, and hips.
- Improves posture and reduces joint pain.
- Releases tension and stiffness in the sides, shoulders, upper back, chest, and hips.
- It may help stimulate digestion and soothe mild stomach discomfort.
- Reduces the risk of slips and falls by improving balance and stability.

ARM SWEEP with KNEE LIFT

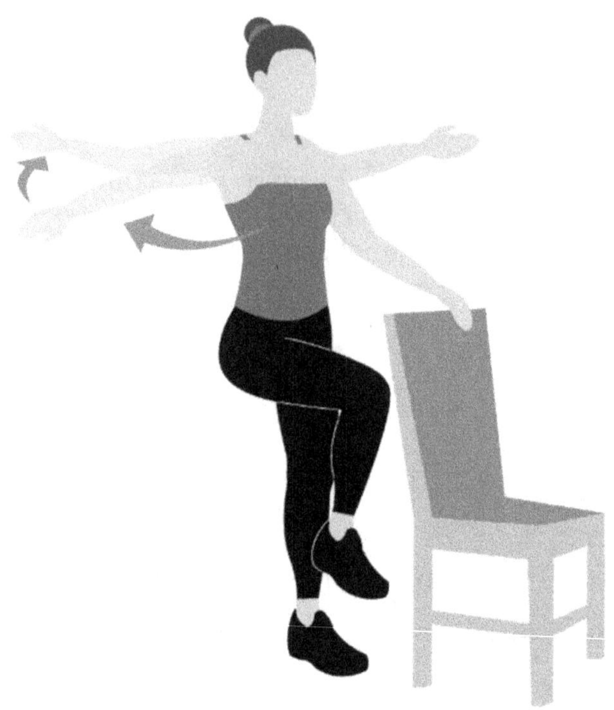

INSTRUCTIONS

1. Stand facing the back of a chair with your left hand on the chair's back.

2. Slowly extend your right arm to the front, lifting your right knee.

3. Slowly sweep your right arm to the right side and then behind you.

4. Sweep the same arm back to the front, keeping it level.

5. Gently stand up straight, then slowly switch sides.

6. Slowly extend your left arm to the front, lifting your left knee.

7. Slowly sweep your left arm to the left side and then behind you.

8. Sweep the same arm back to the front, keeping it level.

9. Continue alternating sides a few times or for as long as it feels good, then gently come to a stop.

ARM SWEEP with KNEE LIFT

Breathing Guide

- Inhale: As you extend your arm to the front and lift your knee.
- Exhale: As you sweep your arm to the side and then behind you.
- Inhale: As you sweep your arm back to the front and lower your knee.

* If the suggested breathing feels challenging or uncomfortable, breathe naturally and easily. As you become more familiar with the pose, you can gradually explore the suggested breathing pattern.

Modifications Guide

- Shoulders feeling stiff? Only move your arm as much as is comfortable.
- Feeling unsteady? Stand hip-width apart, feet flat on the floor.
- Knees feeling stiff? Only bend your knee as much as is comfortable.

Safety Guide

- Move slowly and smoothly. Avoid any sudden or jerky movements.
- Listen to your body. Stop if you feel any discomfort.
- Stand up straight and avoid leaning.

Benefits Guide

- Improves mobility and flexibility in the shoulder, hip, and knee.
- Improves circulation in the arms, legs, and feet, which can help with swelling.
- Reduces the risk of slips and falls by improving balance and stability.
- Improves posture and reduces joint pain.

WARRIOR II

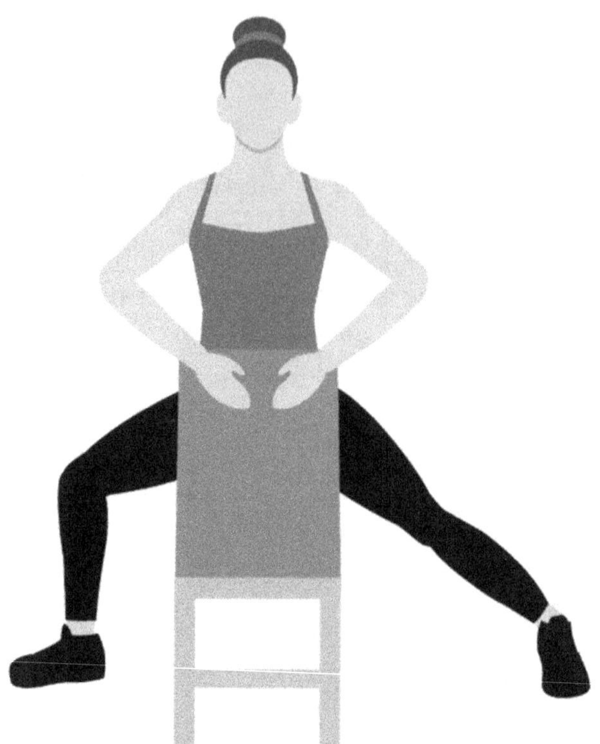

INSTRUCTIONS

1. Stand facing the back of your chair while holding the chair's back with both hands.

2. Slowly extend your left leg to the side with that foot pointing forward.

3. Gently bend your right knee over your ankle with that foot pointing right.

4. Hold this pose for a few breaths, then gently stand up straight.

5. Slowly switch sides.

6. Stand facing the back of your chair while holding the chair's back with both hands.

7. Slowly extend your right leg to the side with that foot pointing forward.

8. Gently bend your left knee over your ankle with that foot pointing left.

9. Continue alternating sides a few times or for as long as it feels good, then gently come to a stop.

WARRIOR II

Breathing Guide

- Inhale: As you extend your leg out to the side.
- Exhale: As you bend the other knee over your ankle.

* If the suggested breathing feels challenging or uncomfortable, breathe naturally and easily. As you become more familiar with the pose, you can gradually explore the suggested breathing pattern.

Modifications Guide

- Hips feeling stiff? Only extend your legs as much as is comfortable.
- Knee feeling stiff? Only bend your knees as much as is comfortable.

Safety Guide

- Move slowly and smoothly. Avoid any sudden or jerky movements.
- Listen to your body. Stop if you feel any discomfort.
- Stand up straight and avoid leaning.
- Don't let your knee go past your toes. Align your bent knee directly over your ankle.
- Engage your core to support your back and maintain balance.

Benefits Guide

- Improves balance and stability by strengthening the legs and ankles.
- Reduces the risk of slips and falls by improving balance and stability.
- Improves mobility and flexibility in the hips and knees.
- Improves mental focus, concentration, and coordination.

TRIANGLE POSE

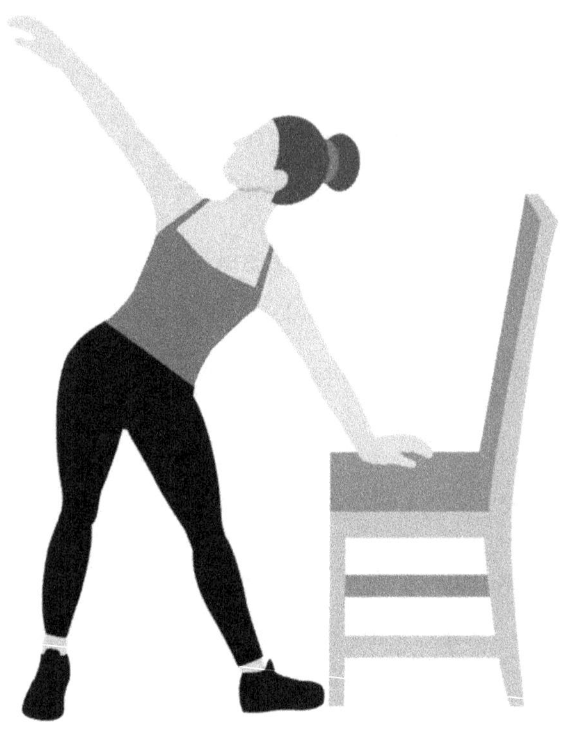

INSTRUCTIONS

1. Stand sideways in front of a chair with your left leg toward the chair.

2. Place your feet shoulder-width apart.

3. Slowly raise your right arm toward the sky.

4. Gently reach for the chair's seat, extending your left arm.

5. Hold this pose for a few breaths, then gently stand up straight.

6. Slowly switch sides.

7. Stand sideways in front of a chair with your right leg toward the chair.

8. Slowly raise your left arm toward the sky.

9. Gently reach for the chair's seat, extending your right arm.

10. Continue alternating sides a few times or for as long as it feels good, then gently come to a stop.

TRIANGLE POSE

Breathing Guide

- Inhale: As you raise your arm toward the sky.
- Exhale: As you reach for the chair's seat with your other hand.

* If the suggested breathing feels challenging or uncomfortable, breathe naturally and easily. As you become more familiar with the pose, you can gradually explore the suggested breathing pattern.

Modifications Guide

- Shoulder feeling stiff? Rest your raised hand on the top of your head.
- Legs feeling stiff? Bend your knees slightly for comfort.
- Feeling unsteady? Stand with your feet wider for better balance.

Safety Guide

- Move slowly and smoothly. Avoid any sudden or jerky movements.
- Listen to your body. Stop if you feel any discomfort.
- Keep your core engaged and avoid rounding your back.
- Don't overstretch. Only reach as far as is comfortable.

Benefits Guide

- Improves mobility and flexibility in the legs, back, and shoulders.
- Improves balance and stability by strengthening the legs and ankles.
- It may help stimulate digestion and soothe mild stomach discomfort.
- Improves mood and reduces stress.
- Reduces the risk of slips and falls by improving balance and stability.

TREE POSE

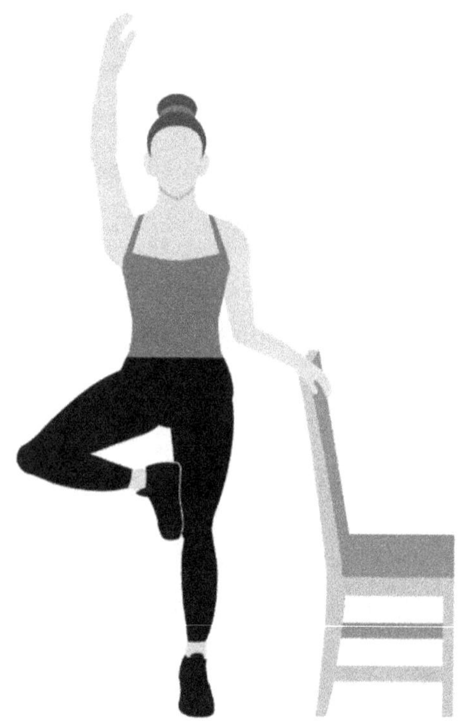

INSTRUCTIONS

1. Stand sideways behind a chair, holding the chair's back with your left hand.

2. Gently place the sole of your right foot on your inner left thigh.

3. Slowly raise your right arm toward the sky.

4. Hold this pose for a few breaths, then gently stand up straight.

5. Slowly switch sides.

6. Stand sideways behind a chair, holding the chair's back with your right hand.

7. Gently place the sole of your left foot on your inner right thigh.

8. Slowly raise your left arm toward the sky.

9. Hold this pose for a few breaths, then gently stand up straight.

10. Continue alternating sides a few times or for as long as it feels good, then gently come to a stop.

TREE POSE

Breathing Guide

- Inhale: As you lift your foot and reach your arm toward the sky.
- Exhale: As you place the sole of your foot on your inner thigh.

* If the suggested breathing feels challenging or uncomfortable, breathe naturally and easily. As you become more familiar with the pose, you can gradually explore the suggested breathing pattern.

Modifications Guide

- Feeling unsteady? Place the sole of your raised foot on your inner calf.
- Feeling unstable? Keep both feet flat on the floor, hip-width apart.
- Shoulder feeling stiff? Rest your raised hand on the top of your head.

Safety Guide

- Move slowly and smoothly. Avoid any sudden or jerky movements.
- Listen to your body. Stop if you feel any discomfort.
- Engage your core to support your back and maintain balance.

Benefits Guide

- Reduces the risk of slips and falls by improving balance and stability.
- Improves mental focus, concentration, and coordination.
- Improves mobility and flexibility in the shoulders, hips, and legs.
- Reduces the risk of slips and falls by strengthening the core, legs, ankles, and feet.

PIGEON POSE

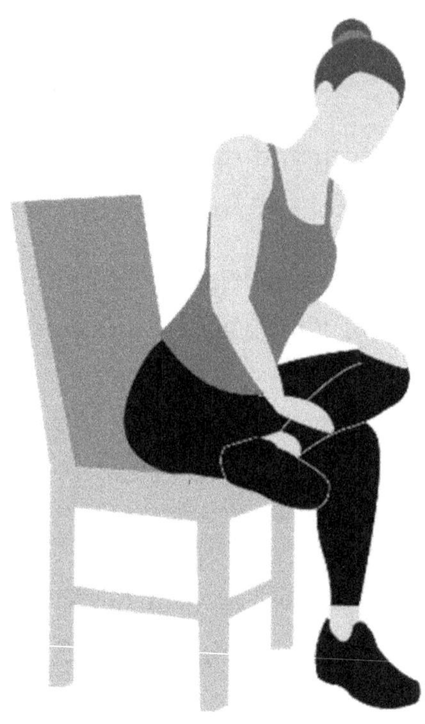

INSTRUCTIONS

1. Sit up straight with your feet flat on the floor.

2. Gently cross your left ankle over your right leg.

3. Rest your hands comfortably on your legs.

4. Slowly lean forward at the hips, keeping your back straight.

5. Hold this pose for a few breaths, then gently sit up straight.

6. Slowly switch legs.

7. Gently cross your right ankle over your left leg.

8. Rest your hands comfortably on your legs.

9. Slowly lean forward at the hips, keeping your back straight.

10. Continue alternating legs a few times or for as long as it feels good, then gently come to a stop.

PIGEON POSE

Breathing Guide

- Inhale: As you sit up straight and prepare to cross your ankle.
- Exhale: As you cross your ankle and lean forward.

* If the suggested breathing feels challenging or uncomfortable, breathe naturally and easily. As you become more familiar with the pose, you can gradually explore the suggested breathing pattern.

Modifications Guide

- Hips feeling stiff? Cross your ankle only where it feels comfortable.
- Knee feeling stiff? Slide your bottom foot forward to lower the height of your crossed ankle.
- Feeling unsteady? Don't lean forward. Sit with your back against the chair's back for support.

Safety Guide

- Move slowly and smoothly. Avoid any sudden or jerky movements.
- Listen to your body. Stop if you feel any discomfort.
- Don't overstretch. Only lean forward as far as is comfortable.

Benefits Guide

- Improves mobility and flexibility in the hips and lower back.
- Releases tension and stiffness in the hips, lower back, glutes, and thighs.
- It may help stimulate digestion and soothe mild stomach discomfort.
- Improves posture and reduces joint pain.
- Improves mood and reduces stress.

Progress in Motion

Congratulations on completing this essential step in your chair yoga journey! By reviewing The Pose Library first, you've laid a strong foundation for success. You've not only familiarized yourself with the poses but also helped your body and mind begin working together even before you've begun to move.

These foundational poses are now part of your personal toolbox—a pocketful of poses, ready to support your routines ahead. Even if some of them seemed challenging or unfamiliar, that's okay; it's all part of the process. The work you've done here will make your practice feel more natural, intuitive, and rewarding as you continue.

My Chair Yoga Journal

Whatever you're thinking or feeling right now, this moment is uniquely yours—it will never happen again. Embrace it! Use the space below to reflect on how you feel, what you're looking forward to, and the things you'll enjoy as you build strength, ease stiffness, and discover more freedom. This journey is all yours, so feel free to make it your own.

____

____

____

____

____

____

____

____

____

Chapter 3

Release Neck & Shoulder Tension

Day 1 Routine: Neck & Shoulders

Today's session focuses on your neck and shoulders. These mindful movements will help you release tension, improve mobility, and increase flexibility naturally.

Most poses can be practiced for up to 2 minutes. Break each pose into short intervals and allow time for switching sides, holding, and resting as needed. This approach keeps the daily routine around 10 minutes, but always focus on moving at a pace that feels safe and comfortable for you.

A Review of The Plan in Practice

The Day 1 Routine is part of a structured program designed to guide your practice step by step. The plan includes 5 daily routines, each featuring 5 carefully chosen poses, practiced weekly across 4 phases. We suggest 5 days of routines followed by 2 rest days, but always listen to your body and rest whenever needed. When you're ready, gradually move toward the full program at a pace that feels right for you.

Each phase builds on the one before it, guiding you week by week toward lasting change. Completing all 4 phases is just the beginning—it sets the stage for a deeper practice and a lifetime of independence. You'll discover more about the phases and challenges as you progress through the book. **Today's session begins now.**

Day 1 Routine Preview: Neck & Shoulders

These five carefully chosen exercises are designed to release stiffness in your neck and shoulders while enhancing mobility and flexibility.

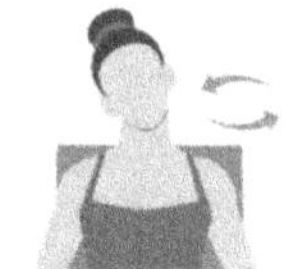

1. Neck Rolls

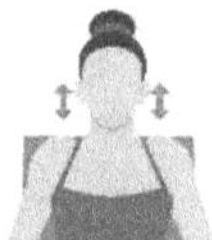

2. Shoulder Shrugs

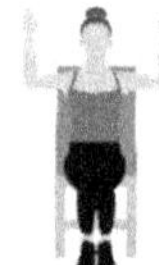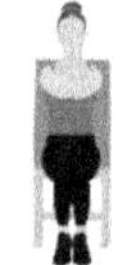

3. Cactus Arms

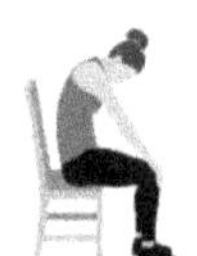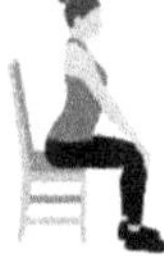

4. Cat-Cow Pose

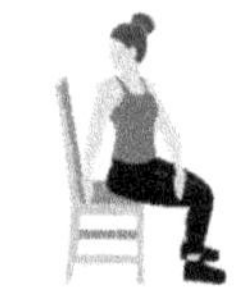

5. Seated Twist

Follow the instructions for each exercise on the following pages—everything you need is right here. If you'd like additional guidance or modifications, you can always refer back to The Pose Library in Chapter 2.

Day 1 Routine
Exercise 1: Neck Rolls

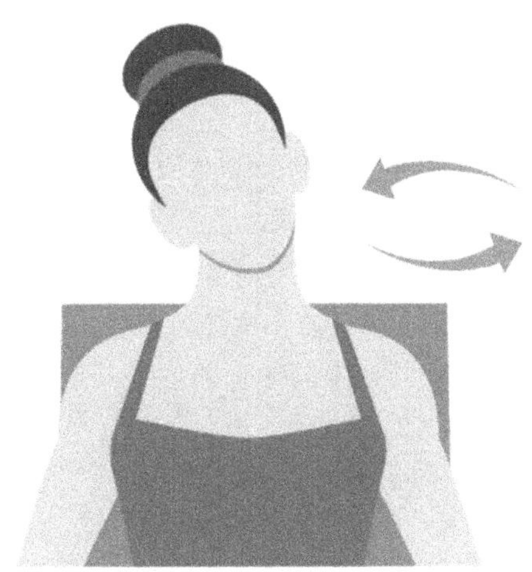

Instructions

1. Sit up straight with your feet flat on the floor.
2. Gently tilt your head to one side, then slowly roll your chin toward your chest.
3. Slowly roll your head to the other side, then back to the center.
4. Gently change directions.
5. Continue alternating directions a few times or for as long as it feels good, then gently come to a stop.

Breathing Guide

- Breathe naturally throughout the movement.

Modification Guide

- Neck feeling stiff? Try gentle side-to-side head tilts instead of full circles.

Safety Guide

- Move slowly and smoothly. Stop if you feel any discomfort.

Benefit Guide

- Releases tension and stiffness in the neck and shoulders.

Pose Guide

- Find more info on this pose in The Pose Library on page 18.

Day 1 Routine
Exercise 2: Shoulder Shrugs

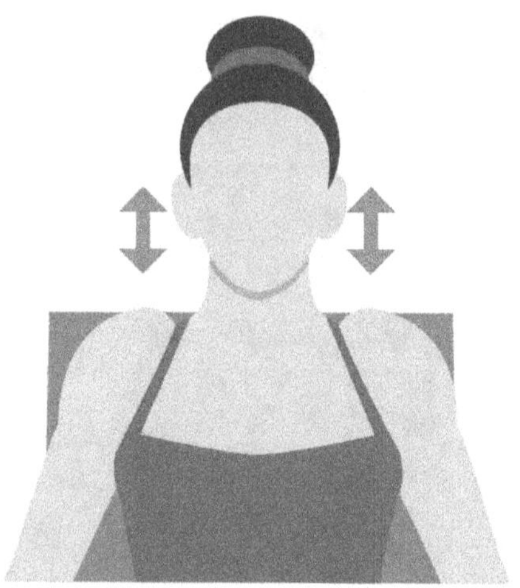

Instructions

1. Sit up straight with your feet flat on the floor.
2. Gently lift your shoulders toward your ears.
3. Slowly lower your shoulders to a natural resting position.
4. Repeat this movement a few times or for as long as it feels good, then gently come to a stop.

Breathing Guide

- Inhale: As you lift your shoulders toward your ears.
- Exhale: As you lower your shoulders to a natural resting position.

Modification Guide

- Shoulders feeling stiff? Only move your shoulders as much as is comfortable.

Safety Guide

- Listen to your body. Stop if you feel any discomfort.

Benefit Guide

- Releases tension and stiffness in the neck and shoulders.

Learn More

- Find more info on this pose in The Pose Library on page 20.

Day 1 Routine
Exercise 3: Cactus Arms

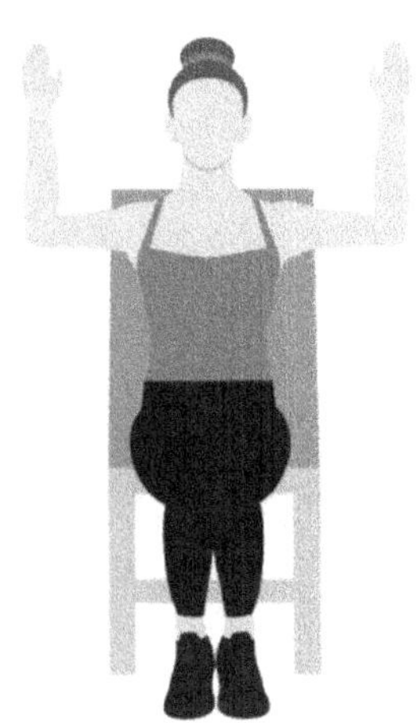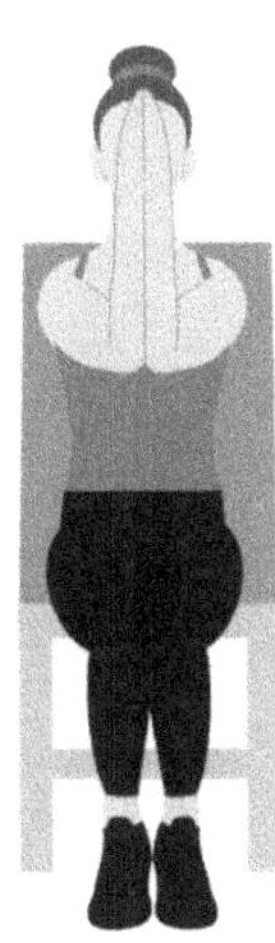

Instructions

1. Sit up straight with your feet flat on the floor.
2. Lift your elbows to your sides in an "L" shape, palms facing forward.
3. Gently bring your forearms together.
4. Slowly open your arms out to your sides.
5. Repeat this movement a few times or for as long as it feels good, then gently come to a stop.

Breathing Guide

- Inhale: As you open your forearms to your sides.
- Exhale: As you bring your forearms together.

Modification Guide

- Shoulders feeling stiff? Only bring your forearms as close together as is comfortable.

Safety Guide

- Listen to your body. Stop if you feel any discomfort.

Benefit Guide

- Reduces tightness in the chest, helping to improve breathing.

Pose Guide

- Find more info on this pose in The Pose Library on page 22.

Day 1 Routine
Exercise 4: Cat Cow Pose

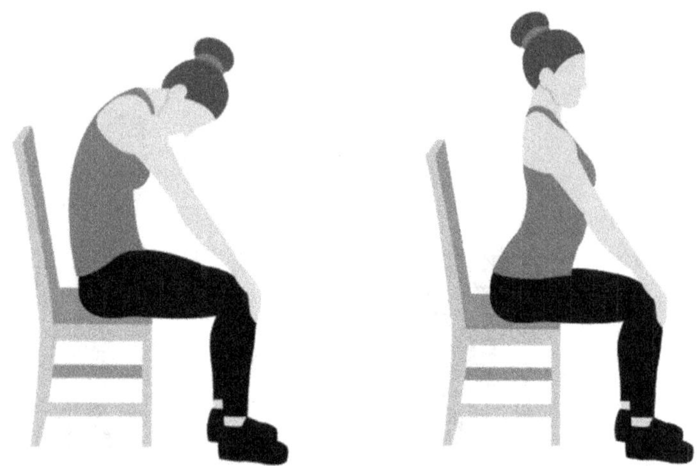

Instructions

1. Sit up straight with your feet flat on the floor.
2. Slowly curl your back like a cat and drop your chin.
3. Hold this pose for a few breaths, then slowly switch poses.
4. Gently lift your chest and dip your lower back like a cow.
5. Hold this pose for a few breaths, then gently sit up straight.
6. Continue alternating poses a few times or for as long as it feels good, then gently come to a stop.

Breathing Guide

- Inhale: As you curl your back like a cat.
- Exhale: As you lift your chest and dip your lower back like a cow.

Modification Guide

- Back feeling stiff? Only arch and dip your back as much as is comfortable.

Safety Guide

- Listen to your body. Stop if you feel any discomfort.

Benefit Guide

- Releases tension and stiffness in your back and shoulders.

Pose Guide

- Find more info on this pose in The Pose Library on page 24.

Day 1 Routine
Exercise 5: Seated Twist

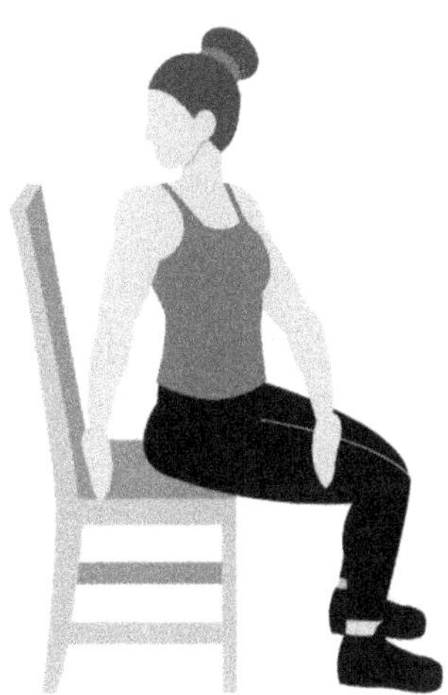

Instructions

1. Sit up straight with your feet flat on the floor.
2. Place your right hand behind you on the chair
3. Place your left hand on your outer right thigh.
4. Gently twist to the right, looking over your right shoulder.
5. Hold this pose for a few breaths, then switch sides.
6. Continue alternating sides a few times or for as long as it feels good, then gently come to a stop.

Breathing Guide

- Inhale: As you sit up straight and prepare to twist.
- Exhale: As you gently twist your body.

Modification Guide

- Back feeling stiff? Only twist your body as much as is comfortable.

Safety Guide

- Listen to your body. Stop if you feel any discomfort.

Benefit Guide

- Releases tension and stiffness in the back, shoulders, and chest.

Pose Guide

- Find more info on this pose in The Pose Library on page 26.

A Mindful Moment

Take a moment to pause, bringing your attention to your neck and shoulders. Notice any new sensations—maybe they feel a bit looser, more open, or warm from today's movements.

Now, let's take a few deep breaths together. Inhale deeply, letting your lungs expand and your body soften. Exhale slowly, releasing any remaining tension with each breath.

Continue this gentle breathing, reflecting on your practice and allowing your body and mind to rest and recover.

Tomorrow, we'll explore new movements to strengthen and relax your arms and hands. Until then, embrace the power of your practice and enjoy the freedom and focus it brings to your day.

My Chair Yoga Journal

Use this space to jot down any reflections, observations, or modifications you'd like to remember from today's practice. This is your personal journey, so feel free to shape it in a way that feels meaningful to you.

Chapter 4

Relieve Stiff Arms & Hands

Day 2 Routine: Arms & Hands

Today's session focuses on your arms and hands. These mindful movements will help you release tension, improve mobility, and increase flexibility naturally.

Remember, most poses can be practiced for up to 2 minutes. Break each pose into short intervals and allow time for switching sides, holding, and resting as needed. This approach keeps the daily routine around 10 minutes, but always focus on moving at a pace that feels safe and comfortable for you.

A Reminder of The Plan in Practice

The Day 2 Routine is part of a structured program designed to guide your practice step by step. The plan includes 5 daily routines, each featuring 5 carefully chosen poses, practiced weekly across 4 phases. We suggest 5 days of routines followed by 2 rest days, but always listen to your body and rest whenever needed. When you're ready, gradually move toward the full program at a pace that feels right for you.

Each phase builds on the one before it, guiding you week by week toward lasting change. Completing all 4 phases is just the beginning—it sets the stage for a deeper practice and a lifetime of celebrations. You'll discover more about the phases and challenges as you progress through the book. **Ready? Let's begin.**

Day 2 Routine Preview: Arms & Hands

These five carefully chosen exercises are designed to relieve stiffness in your arms and hands while enhancing mobility and flexibility.

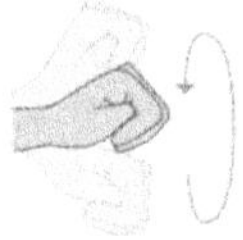

1. Wrist Circles

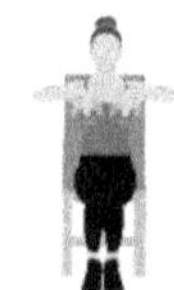

2. Wrist Shakes

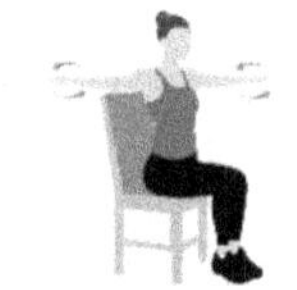

3. Arm Circles

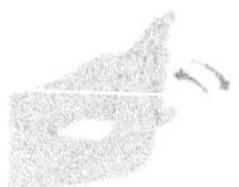

4. Wrist Stretches

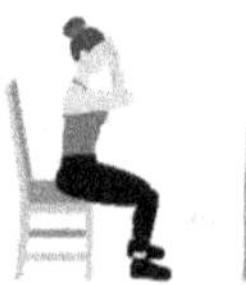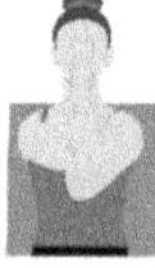

5. Eagle Arms

Follow the instructions for each exercise on the following pages—everything you need is right here. If you'd like additional guidance or modifications, you can always refer back to The Pose Library in Chapter 2.

Day 2 Routine
Exercise 1: Wrist Circles

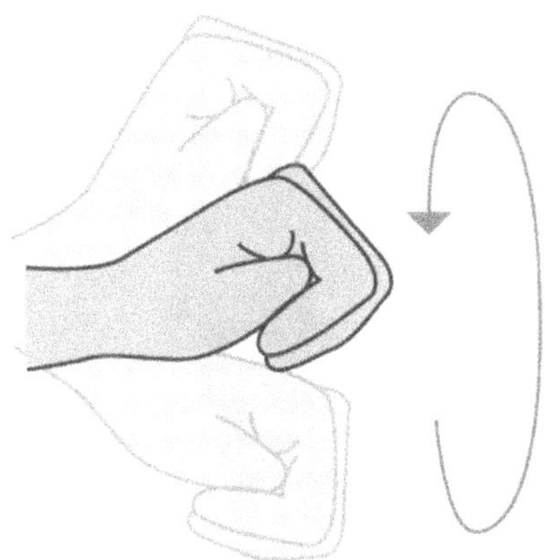

Instructions

1. Sit up straight with your feet flat on the floor.
2. Slowly extend your arms to the front, bending your elbows slightly.
3. Gently make soft, loose fists with your hands.
4. Slowly make circles in one direction with your wrists.
5. Gradually make the circles bigger.
6. Continue for a few breaths, then gently change directions.
7. Continue alternating directions a few times or for as long as it feels good, then gently come to a stop.

Breathing Guide

- Breathe naturally throughout the movement.

Modification Guide

- Wrists feeling stiff? Only circle your wrists as much as is comfortable.

Safety Guide

- Listen to your body. Stop if you feel any discomfort.

Benefit Guide

- Releases tension and stiffness in the hands and wrists.

Pose Guide

- Find more info on this pose in The Pose Library on page 28.

Day 2 Routine
Exercise 2: Wrist Shakes

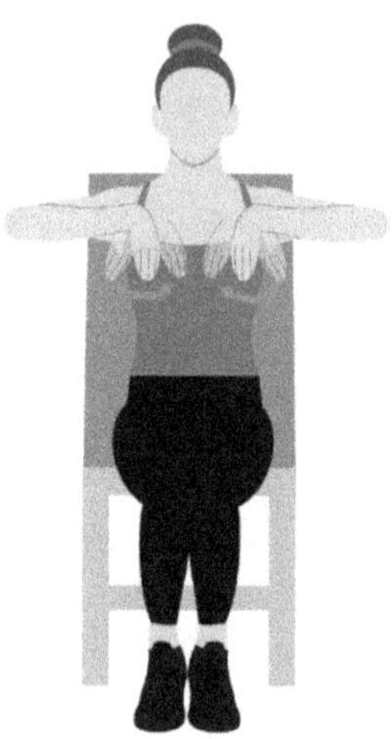

Instructions

1. Sit up straight with your feet flat on the floor.
2. Slowly bend your elbows, lifting your hands and forearms to your chest.
3. Gently shake your hands and wrists from side to side.
4. Continue shaking for a few breaths, then rest your arms comfortably.
5. Repeat this movement a few times or for as long as it feels good, then gently come to a stop.

Breathing Guide

- Breathe naturally and comfortably throughout the exercise.

Modification Guide

- Wrists feeling stiff? Only shake your wrists as much as is comfortable.

Safety Guide

- Listen to your body. Stop if you feel any discomfort.

Benefit Guide

- Releases tension and stiffness in the hands and wrists.

Pose Guide

- Find more info on this pose in The Pose Library on page 30.

Day 2 Routine
Exercise 3: Arm Circles

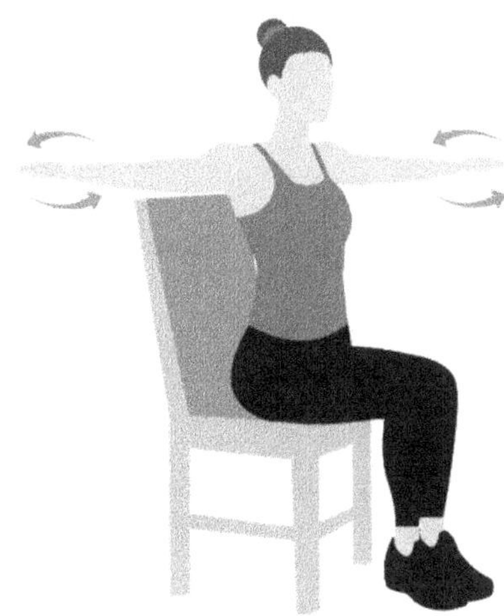

Instructions Guide

1. Sit up straight with your feet flat on the floor.
2. Gently extend your arms to your sides, palms facing down.
3. Slowly make circles with your arms in one direction.
4. Gradually make the circles bigger.
5. Continue for a few breaths, then gently change directions.
6. Continue alternating directions a few times or for as long as it feels good, then gently come to a stop.

Breathing Guide

- Breathe naturally and comfortably throughout the exercise.

Modification Guide

- Shoulders feeling stiff? Only move your arms as much as is comfortable.

Safety Guide

- Listen to your body. Stop if you feel any discomfort.

Benefit Guide

- Releases tension and stiffness in the shoulders and upper back.

Pose Guide

- Find more info on this pose in The Pose Library on page 32.

Day 2 Routine
Exercise 4: Wrist Stretches

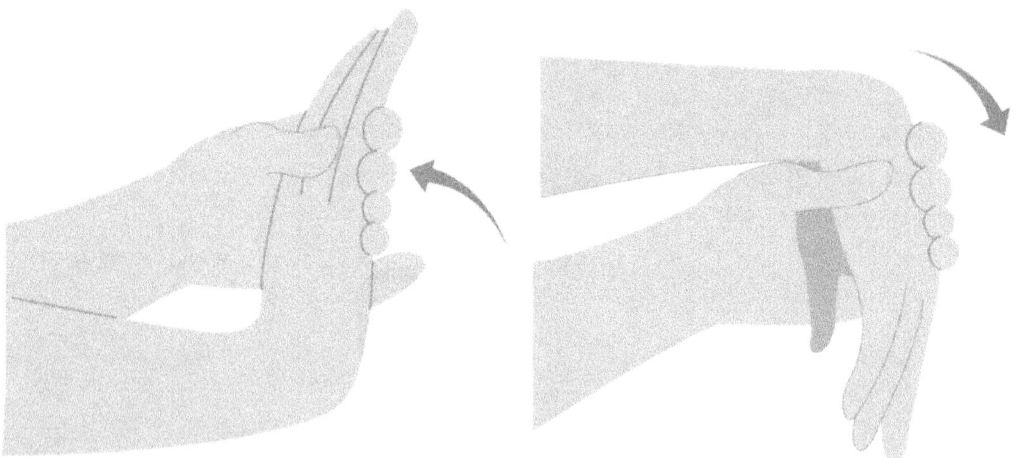

Instructions Guide

1. Sit up straight with your feet flat on the floor.
2. Slowly extend one arm to the front, palm facing down.
3. Gently bend that wrist backward, assisting the bend with the other hand.
4. Hold this pose for a few breaths, then switch directions.
5. Gently bend that wrist forward, assisting the bend with the other hand.
6. Continue alternating directions and arms a few times or for as long as it feels good, then gently come to a stop.

Breathing Guide

- Breathe naturally throughout the movement.

Modification Guide

- Wrists feeling stiff? Only bend your wrist as much as is comfortable.

Safety Guide

- Listen to your body. Stop if you feel any discomfort.

Benefit Guide

- Releases tension and stiffness in the hands and wrists.

Pose Guide

- Find more info on this pose in The Pose Library on page 34.

Day 2 Routine
Exercise 5: Eagle Arms

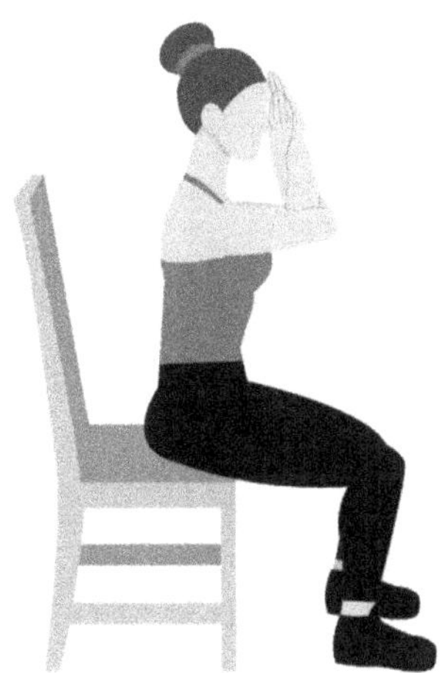 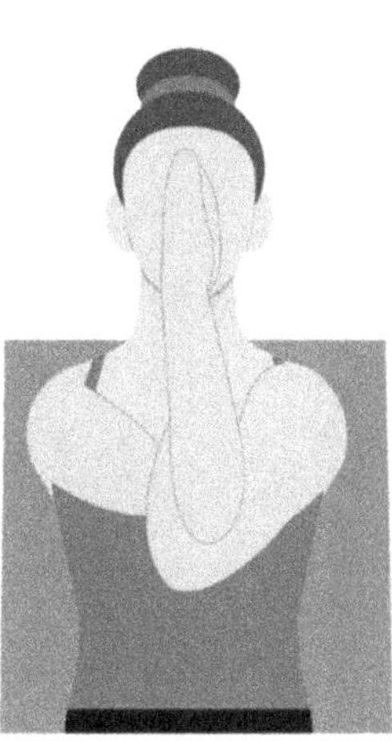

Instructions Guide

1. Sit up straight with your feet flat on the floor.
2. Slowly extend your arms and cross your left elbow over your right.
3. Gently bend your elbows up and crisscross your forearms.
4. Slowly bring the backs of your hands together and lift your elbows.
5. Hold this pose for a few breaths, then slowly switch sides.
6. Continue alternating arms a few times or for as long as it feels good, then gently come to a stop.

Breathing Guide

- Inhale: As you extend your arms and cross your elbows.
- Exhale: As you bend your elbows and crisscross your forearms.

Modification Guide

- Shoulders feeling stiff? Give yourself a big hug instead, reaching your arms across your chest and holding the opposite shoulders.

Safety Guide

- Listen to your body. Stop if you feel any discomfort.

Benefit Guide

- Releases tension and stiffness in the shoulders, upper back, and neck.

Pose Guide

- Find more info on this pose in The Pose Library on page 36.

A Mindful Moment

Take a moment to pause, bringing your attention to your arms and hands. Notice any new sensations—maybe they're feeling refreshed, loose, or energized from today's movements.

Now, let's take a few deep breaths together. Inhale deeply, letting your lungs expand and your body soften. Exhale slowly, releasing any remaining tension with each breath.

Continue this gentle breathing, reflecting on your practice and allowing your body and mind to rest and recover.

Tomorrow, we'll explore new movements to strengthen and relax your legs and feet. Until then, embrace the power of your practice and enjoy the freedom and focus it brings to the rest of your day.

My Chair Yoga Journal

Use this space to jot down any reflections, observations, or modifications you'd like to remember from today's practice. This is your personal journey, so feel free to shape it in a way that feels meaningful to you.

____

____

____

____

____

____

Chapter 5

Rescue Tired Legs & Feet

Day 3 Routine: Legs & Feet

Today's session focuses on your legs and feet. These mindful movements will help you release stiffness, improve mobility, and increase flexibility naturally.

Remember, most poses can be practiced for up to 2 minutes. Break each pose into short intervals and allow time for switching sides, holding, and resting as needed. This approach keeps the daily routine around 10 minutes, but always focus on moving at a pace that feels safe and comfortable for you.

A Reminder of The Plan in Practice

The Day 3 Routine is part of a structured program designed to guide your practice step by step. The plan includes 5 daily routines, each featuring 5 carefully chosen poses, practiced weekly across 4 phases. We suggest 5 days of routines followed by 2 rest days, but always listen to your body and rest whenever needed. When you're ready, gradually move toward the full program at a pace that feels right for you.

Each phase builds on the one before it, guiding you week by week toward lasting change. Completing all 4 phases is just the beginning—it sets the stage for a deeper practice and a lifetime of confidence. You'll discover more about the phases and challenges as you progress through the book. **Now, let's begin today's session.**

Day 3 Routine Preview: Legs & Feet

These five carefully chosen exercises are designed to rescue tired legs and feet while enhancing mobility and flexibility.

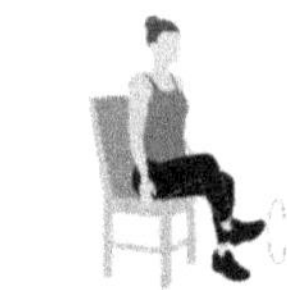

1. Ankle Circles

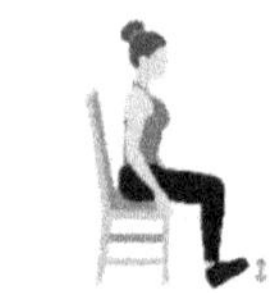

2. Toe Raises

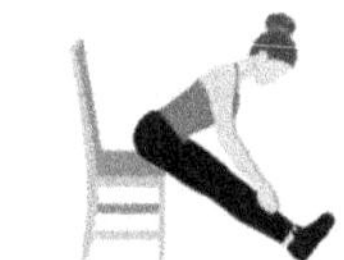

3. Forward Bend

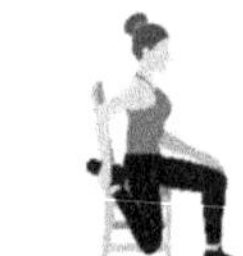

4. Quad Stretch

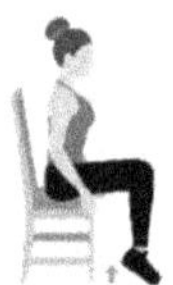

6. Heel Raises

Follow the instructions for each exercise on the following pages—everything you need is right here. If you'd like additional guidance or modifications, you can always refer back to The Pose Library in Chapter 2.

Day 3 Routine
Exercise 1: Ankle Circles

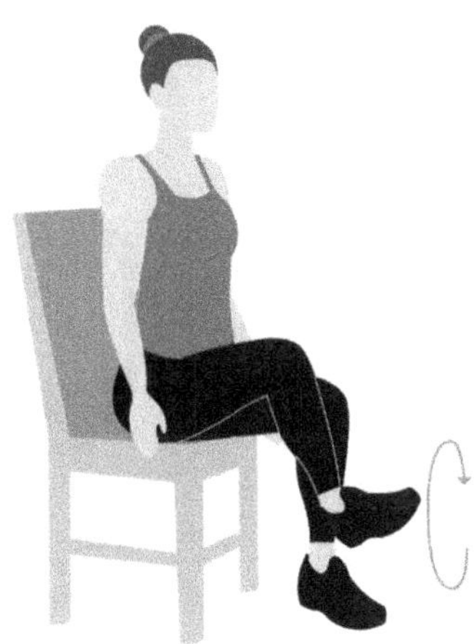

Instructions

1. Sit up straight with your feet flat on the floor.
2. Slowly lift your right foot off the floor.
3. Gently make circles with that ankle, gradually making them bigger.
4. Continue for a few breaths, then change directions.
5. Continue for a few breaths, then lower your right foot.
6. Slowly switch sides, repeating the circles with your left ankle.
7. Continue alternating directions and sides a few times or for as long as it feels good, then gently come to a stop.

Breathing Guide

- Breathe naturally throughout the movement.

Modification Guide

- Feet feeling stiff? Only make the circles as big as is comfortable.

Safety Guide

- Listen to your body. Stop if you feel any discomfort.

Benefit Guide

- Releases tension and stiffness in the ankles and feet.

Pose Guide

- Find more info on this pose in The Pose Library on page 38.

Day 3 Routine
Exercise 2: Toe Raises

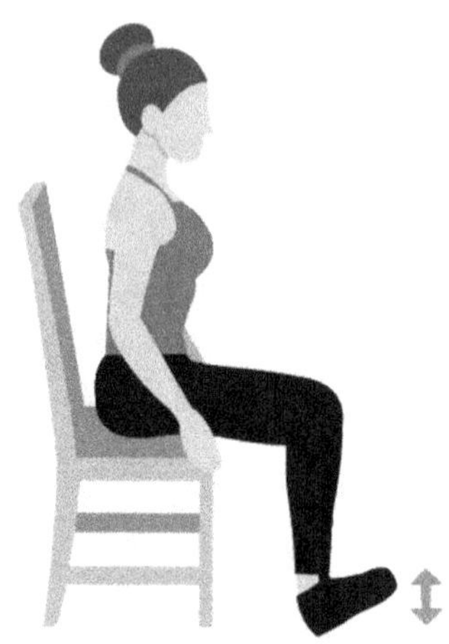

Instructions

1. Sit up straight with your feet flat on the floor.
2. Slowly lift your toes, keeping your heels on the floor.
3. Hold this pose for a few breaths.
4. Slowly lower your toes until both feet are flat on the floor.
5. Repeat this movement a few times or for as long as it feels good, then gently come to a stop.

Breathing Guide

- Inhale: As you lift your toes.
- Exhale: As you lower your toes.

Modification Guide

- Ankles feeling stiff? Only lift your toes as much as is comfortable.

Safety Guide

- Listen to your body. Stop if you feel any discomfort.

Benefit Guide

- Releases tension and stiffness in the ankles and feet.

Pose Guide

- Find more info on this pose in The Pose Library on page 40.

Day 3 Routine
Exercise 3: Forward Bend

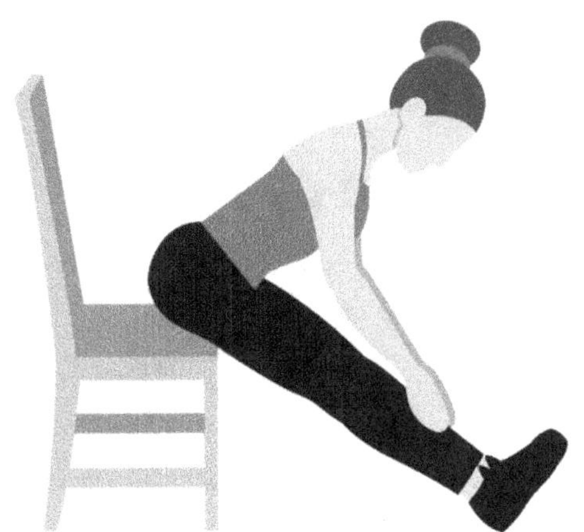

Instructions

1. Sit up straight with your feet flat on the floor.
2. Gently extend your legs, keeping your heels on the floor.
3. Slowly bend forward from your hips, keeping your back straight.
4. Gently reach your hands toward your ankles, extending your arms.
5. Hold this pose for a few breaths, then slowly sit up straight.
6. Gently wiggle your arms, legs, and feet to release tension.
7. Repeat this movement a few times or for as long as it feels good, then gently come to a stop.

Breathing Guide

- Inhale: As you sit up straight and prepare to bend forward.
- Exhale: As you bend forward.

Modification Guide

- Back feeling stiff? Only bend forward as far as is comfortable.

Safety Guide

- Listen to your body. Stop if you feel any discomfort.

Benefit Guide

- Releases tension and stiffness in the lower back, shoulders, and hips.

Pose Guide

- Find more info on this pose in The Pose Library on page 42.

Day 3 Routine
Exercise 4: Quad Stretch

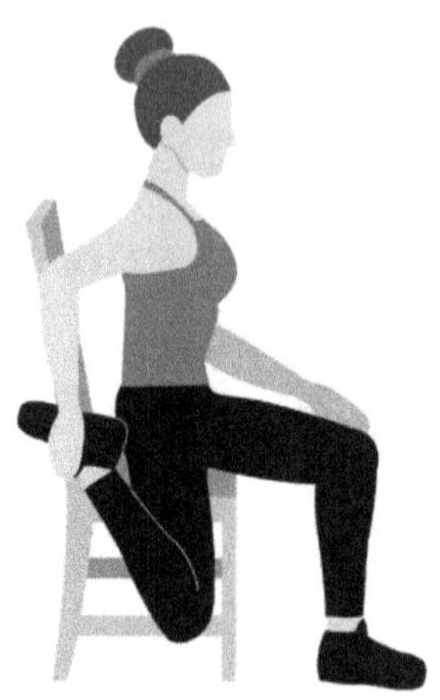

Instructions

1. Sit up straight with your feet flat on the floor.
2. Place your left hand on your left knee.
3. Slowly bend your right knee, bringing that foot behind you.
4. Gently pull your right foot toward your right hip.
5. Hold this pose for a few breaths, then slowly switch sides.
6. Continue alternating sides a few times or for as long as it feels good, then gently come to a stop.

Breathing Guide

- Inhale: As you sit up straight and prepare to bend your knee.
- Exhale: As you pull your foot toward your hip.

Modification Guide

- Knee feeling stiff? Only bend your knee as much as is comfortable.

Safety Guide

- Listen to your body. Stop if you feel any discomfort.

Benefit Guide

- Releases tension and stiffness in the knees and legs

Pose Guide

- Find more info on this pose in The Pose Library on page 44.

Day 3 Routine
Exercise 5: Heel Raises

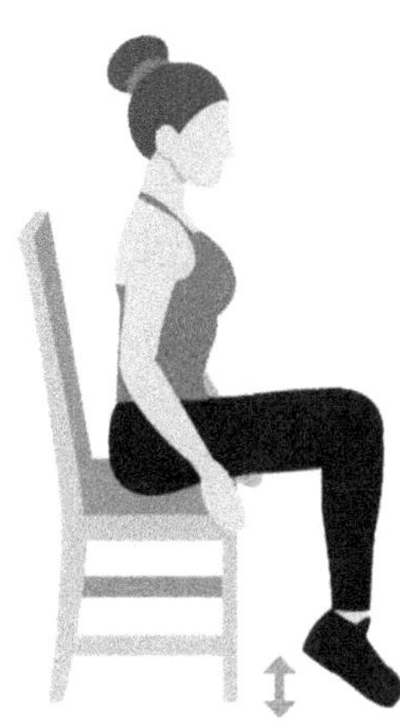

Instructions

1. Sit up straight with your feet flat on the floor.
2. Find a comfortable place to rest your hands.
3. Lift your heels, keeping your toes on the floor.
4. Hold this pose for a few breaths.
5. Slowly lower your heels until both feet are flat on the floor.
6. Continue this movement a few times or for as long as it feels good, then gently come to a stop.

Breathing Guide

- Inhale: As you lift your heels.
- Exhale: As you lower your heels.

Modification Guide

- Feet feeling stiff? Only lift your heels as much as is comfortable.

Safety Guide

- Listen to your body. Stop if you feel any discomfort.

Benefit Guide

- Releases tension and stiffness in the calves, ankles, and feet.

Pose Guide

- Find more info on this pose in The Pose Library on page 46.

A Mindful Moment

Take a moment to pause, bringing your attention to your legs and feet. Notice any new sensations—maybe they feel a little shaky, slightly tender, or even a tiny bit tingly from today's movements.

Now, let's take a few deep breaths together. Inhale deeply, letting your lungs expand and your body soften. Exhale slowly, releasing any remaining tension with each breath.

Continue this gentle breathing, reflecting on your practice and allowing your body and mind to rest and recover.

Tomorrow, we'll explore new movements to strengthen and relax your back and spine. Until then, embrace the power of your practice and enjoy the freedom and focus it brings to your day.

My Chair Yoga Journal

Use this space to jot down any reflections, observations, or modifications you'd like to remember from today's practice. This is your personal journey, so feel free to shape it in a way that feels meaningful to you.

____

____

____

____

____

____

____

Chapter 6

Reduce Back & Spine Pain

Day 4 Routine: Back & Spine

Today's session focuses on your back and spine. These mindful movements will help you release tension, improve mobility, and increase flexibility naturally.

Remember, most poses can be practiced for up to 2 minutes. Break each pose into short intervals and allow time for switching sides, holding, and resting as needed. This approach keeps the daily routine around 10 minutes, but always focus on moving at a pace that feels safe and comfortable for you.

A Reminder of The Plan in Practice

The Day 4 Routine is part of a structured program designed to guide your practice step by step. The plan includes 5 daily routines, each featuring 5 carefully chosen poses, practiced weekly across 4 phases. We suggest 5 days of routines followed by 2 rest days, but always listen to your body and rest whenever needed. When you're ready, gradually move toward the full program at a pace that feels right for you.

Each phase builds on the one before it, guiding you week by week toward lasting change. Completing all 4 phases is just the beginning—it sets the stage for a deeper practice and a lifetime of freedom. You'll discover more about the phases and challenges as you progress through the book. **Welcome to today's session.**

Day 4 Routine Preview: Back & Spine

These five carefully chosen exercises are designed to reduce back and spine pain while enhancing mobility and flexibility.

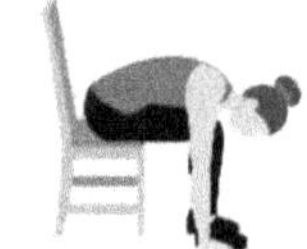

1. Forward Fold

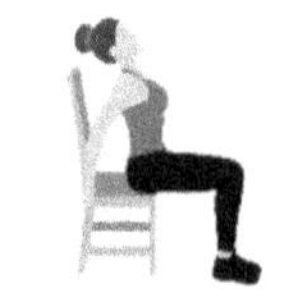

2. Cobra Pose

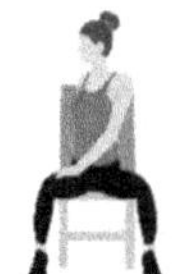

3. Wide-Legged Twist

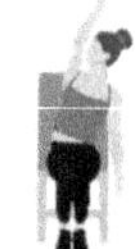

4. Side Stretches

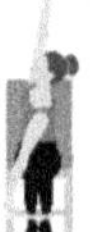

5. Extended Side Angle Pose

Follow the instructions for each exercise on the following pages—everything you need is right here. If you'd like additional guidance or modifications, you can always refer back to The Pose Library in Chapter 2.

Day 4 Routine
Exercise 1: Forward Fold

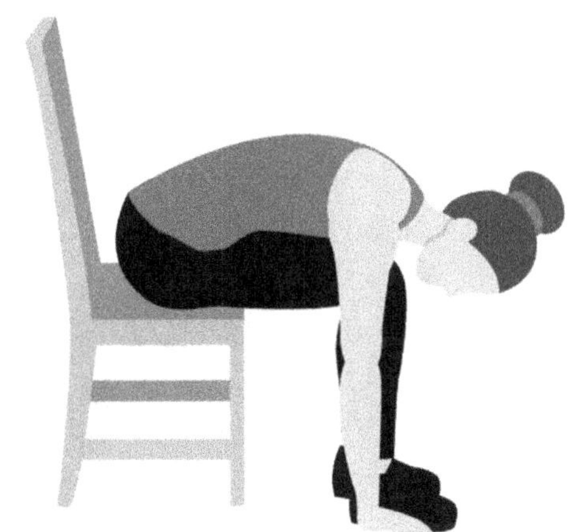

Instructions

1. Sit up straight with your feet flat on the floor.
2. Slowly bend forward from your hips, bringing your chest toward your legs.
3. Gently reach your hands toward the floor, extending your arms.
4. Hold this pose for a few breaths, then slowly sit up straight.
5. Continue this movement a few times or for as long as it feels good, then gently come to a stop.

Breathing Guide

- Inhale: As you sit up straight and prepare to fold forward.
- Exhale: As you fold forward.

Modification Guide

- Back feeling stiff? Only fold forward as much as is comfortable.

Safety Guide

- Listen to your body. Stop if you feel any discomfort.

Benefit Guide

- Releases tension and stiffness in the lower back, shoulders, and hips.

Pose Guide

- Find more info on this pose in The Pose Library on page 48.

Day 4 Routine
Exercise 2: Cobra Pose

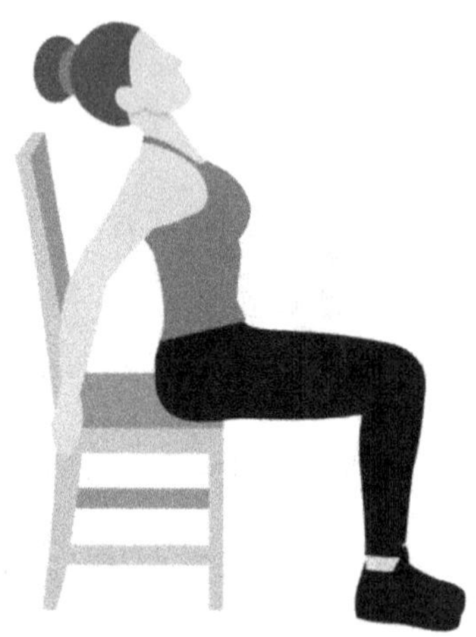

Instructions

1. Sit up straight with your feet flat on the floor.
2. Gently place your hands behind you on the chair.
3. Slowly arch your upper back and lift your chest.
4. Gently tilt your chin upward.
5. Hold this pose for a few breaths, then gently sit up straight.
6. Repeat this movement a few times or for as long as it feels good, then gently come to a stop.

Breathing Guide

- Inhale: As you arch your back and lift your chest and chin.
- Exhale: As you straighten your back and lower your chest and chin.

Modification Guide

- Back feeling stiff? Only arch your back as much as is comfortable.

Safety Guide

- Listen to your body. Stop if you feel any discomfort.

Benefit Guide

- Releases tension and stiffness in the upper back, chest, shoulders, and neck.

Pose Guide

- Find more info on this pose in The Pose Library on page 50.

Day 4 Routine
Exercise 3: Wide-Legged Twist

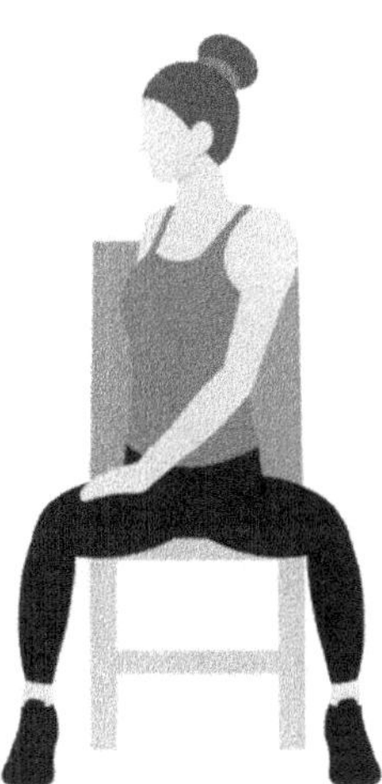

Instructions

1. Sit up straight with your feet flat on the floor.
2. Keep your feet wide with your knees over your ankles.
3. Place your right hand behind you on the chair.
4. Place your left hand on your outer right thigh.
5. Gently turn your body to the right and look over your right shoulder.
6. Hold this pose for a few breaths, then slowly switch sides.
7. Continue alternating sides a few times or for as long as it feels good, then gently come to a stop.

Breathing Guide

- Inhale: As you sit up straight and prepare to turn your body.
- Exhale: As you turn your body.

Modification Guide

- Back feeling stiff? Only turn as much as is comfortable.

Safety Guide

- Listen to your body. Stop if you feel any discomfort.

Benefit Guide

- Releases tension and stiffness in the back, shoulders, sides, and hips.

Pose Guide

- Find more info on this pose in The Pose Library on page 52.

Day 4 Routine
Exercise 4: Side Stretches

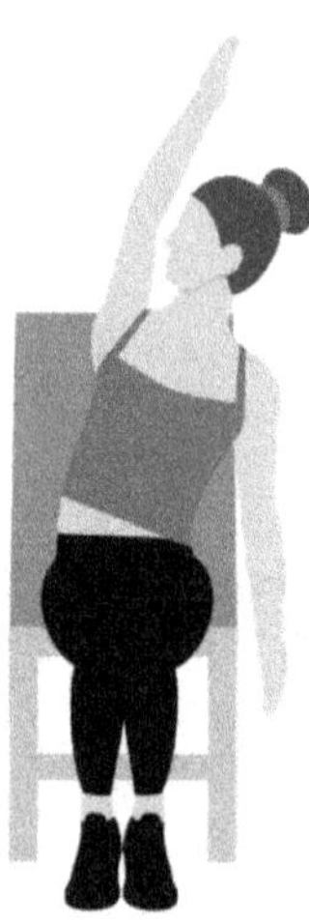

Instructions

1. Sit up straight with your feet flat on the floor.
2. Slowly raise your right arm toward the sky with your palm facing inward.
3. Gently reach your left arm downward, bending your body to the left.
4. Hold this pose for a few breaths, then slowly switch sides.
5. Continue alternating sides a few times or for as long as it feels good, then gently come to a stop.

Breathing Guide

- Inhale: As you reach your raised arm toward the sky.
- Exhale: As you bend your body to the side.

Modification Guide

- Sides feeling stiff? Only bend your body as much as is comfortable.

Safety Guide

- Listen to your body. Stop if you feel any discomfort.

Benefit Guide

- Releases tension and stiffness in the sides, shoulders, upper back, and hips.

Pose Guide

- Find more info on this pose in The Pose Library on page 54.

Day 4 Routine
Exercise 5: Extended Side Angle Pose

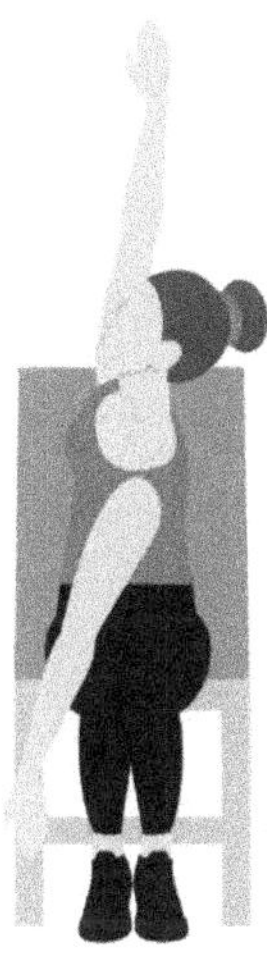

Instructions

1. Sit up straight with your feet flat on the floor.
2. Slowly raise your right arm toward the sky, turning gently to the right.
3. Slowly reach your left hand down toward the outside of your right foot.
4. Hold this pose for a few breaths, then slowly switch sides.
5. Continue alternating sides a few times or for as long as it feels good, then gently come to a stop.

Breathing Guide

- Inhale: As you reach your raised arm toward the sky.
- Exhale: As you reach your lower arm toward the floor.

Modification Guide

- Back feeling stiff? Only turn your body as much as is comfortable.

Safety Guide

- Listen to your body. Stop if you feel any discomfort.

Benefit Guide

- Releases tension and stiffness in the sides, shoulders, upper back, chest, and hips.

Pose Guide

- Find more info on this pose in The Pose Library on page 56.

A Mindful Moment

Take a moment to pause and bring your attention to your back and spine. Notice any new sensations—perhaps your posture feels straighter, your spine longer, or maybe you feel a little taller from today's movements.

Now, let's take a few deep breaths together. Inhale deeply, letting your lungs expand and your body soften. Exhale slowly, releasing any remaining tension with each breath.

Continue this gentle breathing, reflecting on your practice and allowing your body and mind to rest and recover.

Tomorrow, we'll explore new movements that focus on improving your breathing and balance. Until then, embrace the power of your practice and enjoy the freedom and focus it brings to your day.

My Chair Yoga Journal

Use this space to jot down any reflections, observations, or modifications you'd like to remember from today's practice. This is your personal journey, so feel free to shape it in a way that feels meaningful to you.

Chapter 7

Restore Breath & Balance

Day 5 Routine: Breath & Balance

Today's session focuses on your breath and balance. These mindful movements will help you release tension, improve mobility, and increase flexibility naturally.

Remember, most poses can be practiced for up to 2 minutes. Break each pose into short intervals and allow time for switching sides, holding, and resting as needed. This approach keeps the daily routine around 10 minutes, but always focus on moving at a pace that feels safe and comfortable for you.

A Reminder of The Plan in Practice

The Day 5 Routine is part of a structured program designed to guide your practice step by step. The plan includes 5 daily routines, each featuring 5 carefully chosen poses, practiced weekly across 4 phases. We suggest 5 days of routines followed by 2 rest days, but always listen to your body and rest whenever needed. When you're ready, gradually move toward the full program at a pace that feels right for you.

Each phase builds on the one before it, guiding you week by week toward lasting change. Completing all 4 phases is just the beginning—it sets the stage for a deeper practice and a lifetime of wellness. You'll discover more about the phases and challenges as you progress through the book. **Enjoy today's session.**

Day 5 Routine: Breath and Balance

These five carefully chosen exercises are designed to restore breath and balance while enhancing mobility and flexibility.

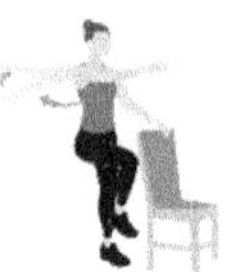

1. Arm Sweep with Knee Lift

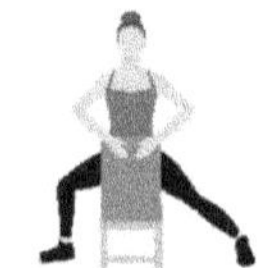

2. Warrior II

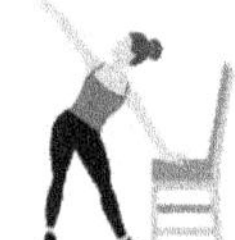

3. Triangle Pose

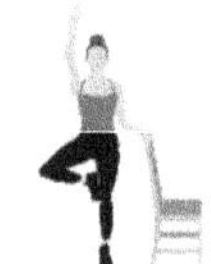

4. Tree Pose

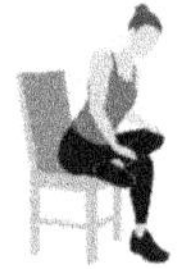

5. Pigeon Pose

Follow the instructions for each exercise on the following pages—everything you need is right here. If you'd like additional guidance or modifications, you can always refer back to The Pose Library in Chapter 2.

Day 5 Routine
Exercise 1: Arm Sweep with Knee Lift

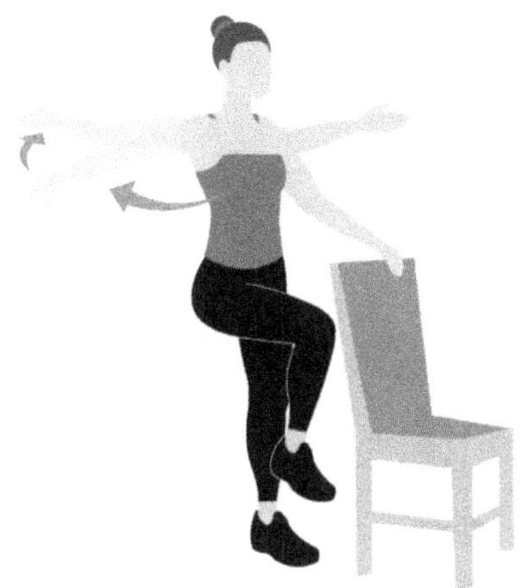

Instructions

1. Stand facing the back of a chair, holding the chair with your left hand.
2. Slowly extend your right arm to the front and raise your right knee.
3. Slowly sweep your right arm to the right side and then behind you.
4. Sweep your right arm back to the front, keeping it level.
5. Gently lower your right arm and knee, then slowly switch sides.
6. Continue alternating sides a few times or for as long as it feels good, then gently come to a stop.

Breathing Guide

- Inhale: As you extend your arm to the front and lift your knee.
- Exhale: As you sweep your arm to the side and then behind you.
- Inhale: As you sweep your arm back to the front and lower your knee.

Modification Guide

- Feeling unsteady? Stand with both feet flat on the floor.

Safety Guide

- Listen to your body. Stop if you feel any discomfort.

Benefit Guide

- Reduces the risk of slips and falls by improving balance and stability.

Pose Guide

- Find more info on this pose in The Pose Library on page 58.

Day 5 Routine
Exercise 2: Warrior II

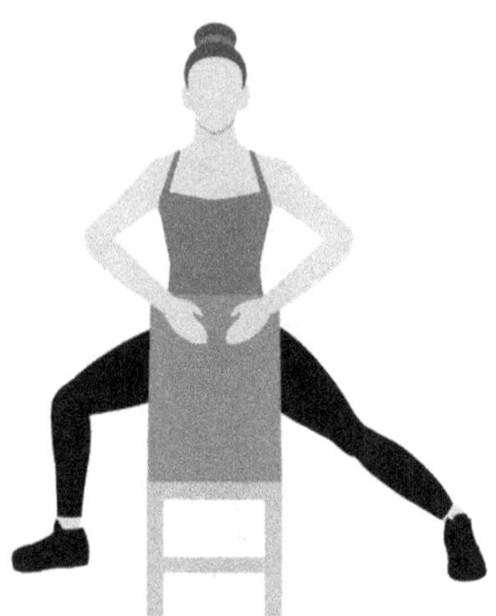

Instructions

1. Stand behind a chair, holding the top of the chair's back with both hands.
2. Slowly extend your left leg to the side, pointing that foot forward.
3. Bend your right knee over your ankle, pointing that foot to the right.
4. Hold this pose for a few breaths, then gently stand up straight.
5. Slowly switch sides.
6. Continue alternating sides a few times or for as long as it feels good, then gently come to a stop.

Breathing Guide

- Inhale: As you extend your leg out to the side.
- Exhale: As you bend the other knee over your ankle.

Modification Guide

- Hips feeling stiff? Only extend your legs as much as is comfortable.

Safety Guide

- Listen to your body. Stop if you feel any discomfort.

Benefit Guide

- Reduces the risk of slips and falls by improving balance and stability.

Pose Guide

- Find more info on this pose in The Pose Library on page 60.

Day 5 Routine
Exercise 3: Triangle Pose

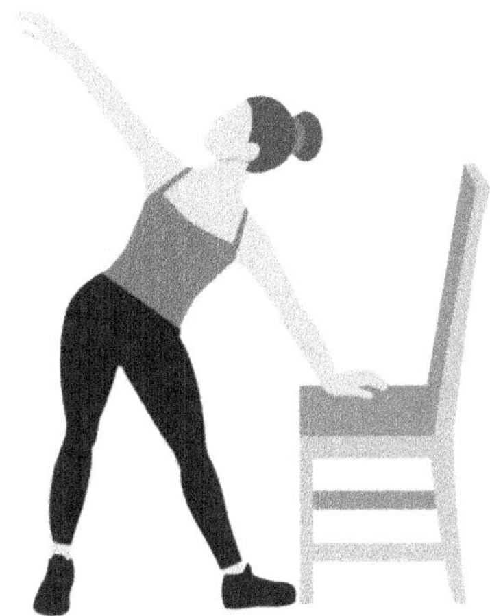

Instructions

1. Stand sideways in front of a chair with your left leg toward the chair.
2. Place your feet hip-width apart and flat on the floor.
3. Slowly raise your right arm toward the sky.
4. Gently reach for the chair's seat with your left hand, extending your arm.
5. Hold this pose for a few breaths, then slowly switch sides.
6. Continue alternating sides a few times or for as long as it feels good, then gently come to a stop.

Breathing Guide

- Inhale: As you raise your arm toward the sky.
- Exhale: As you reach for the chair's seat with your other hand.

Modification Guide

- Legs feeling stiff? Bend your knees slightly for comfort.

Safety Guide

- Listen to your body. Stop if you feel any discomfort.

Benefit Guide

- Reduces the risk of slips and falls by improving balance and stability.

Pose Guide

- Find more info on this pose in The Pose Library on page 62.

Day 5 Routine
Exercise 4: Tree Pose

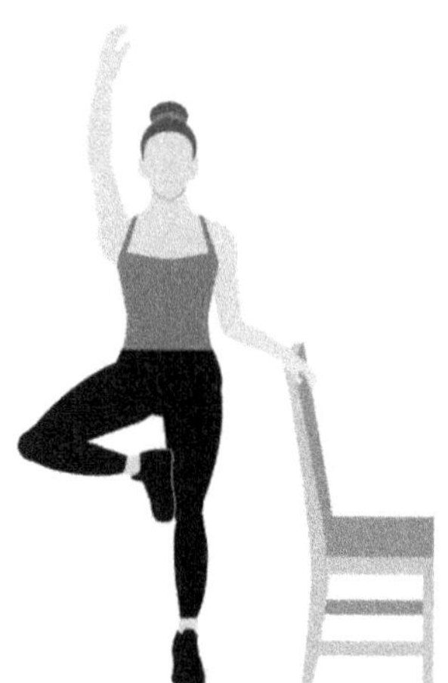

Instructions

1. Stand sideways behind a chair, holding the chair's back with your left hand.
2. Gently place the sole of your right foot on your inner left thigh or calf.
3. Slowly raise your right arm toward the sky, keeping your back straight.
4. Hold this pose for a few breaths, then gently stand up straight.
5. Slowly switch sides.
6. Continue alternating sides a few times or for as long as it feels good, then gently come to a stop.

Breathing Guide

- Inhale: As you lift your foot and reach your arm toward the sky.
- Exhale: As you place the sole of your foot on your inner thigh or calf.

Modification Guide

- Feeling unstable? Keep both feet flat on the floor.

Safety Guide

- Listen to your body. Stop if you feel any discomfort.

Benefit Guide

- Reduces the risk of slips and falls by improving balance and stability.

Pose Guide

- Find more info on this pose in The Pose Library on page 64.

Day 5 Routine
Exercise 5: Pigeon Pose

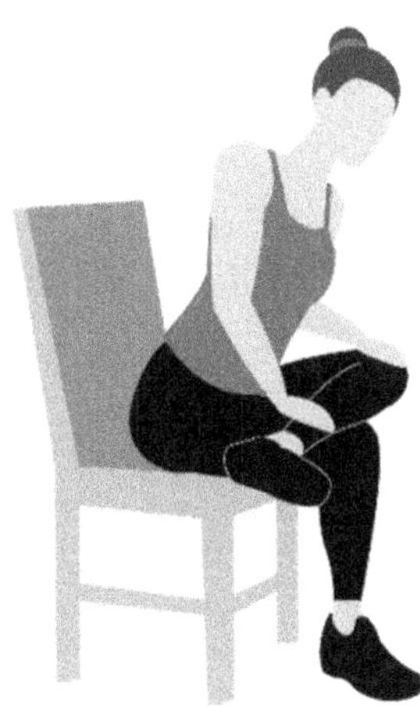

Instructions

1. Sit up straight with your feet flat on the floor.
2. Gently cross your left ankle over your right leg.
3. Rest your hands comfortably on your legs.
4. Slowly lean forward at the hips, keeping your back straight.
5. Hold this pose for a few breaths, then slowly switch legs.
6. Continue alternating sides a few times or for as long as it feels good, then gently come to a stop.

Breathing Guide

- Inhale: As you sit up straight and prepare to cross your ankle.
- Exhale: As you cross your ankle and lean forward.

Modification Guide

- Hips feeling stiff? Only cross your ankle where it feels comfortable.

Safety Guide

- Listen to your body. Stop if you feel any discomfort.

Benefit Guide

- Releases tension and stiffness in the hips, lower back, glutes, and thighs.

Pose Guide

- Find more info on this pose in The Pose Library on page 66.

A Mindful Moment

Pause for a moment and focus on your breath and body. Notice any new sensations—perhaps you feel more open, energized, or focused after today's movements.

Now, let's take a few deep breaths together. Inhale deeply, allowing your body to soften as your lungs expand. Exhale slowly, releasing any remaining tension with each breath.

Continue this gentle breathing, reflecting on your practice and allowing your body and mind to rest and recover.

Tomorrow, we'll explore how to combine these foundational poses into a fulfilling 28-day practice, guiding you toward lifelong independence and relief from aches and pains. Until then, embrace the strength of your practice and enjoy the freedom and focus it brings to your day.

My Chair Yoga Journal

Use this space to jot down any reflections, observations, or modifications you'd like to remember from today's practice. This is your personal journey, so feel free to shape it in a way that feels meaningful to you.

____

____

____

____

____

____

Chapter 8

The Chair Yoga Challenge

The Power of Mindful Movement

Welcome! By choosing this journey, you've taken an incredible step forward, and we're happy you're here. You've joined millions who have embraced this ancient wisdom—now supported by science—to reduce pain, improve mobility, and reclaim their lives. This is more than just a practice; it's a path to lasting relief, renewed freedom, and a stronger connection with yourself.

Pause and reflect on how far you've come. Honor it. Breathe deeply, and recognize the strength, resilience, and commitment that brought you here. Milestones like this deserve to be celebrated. You deserve to be celebrated. Together, we'll build on this momentum, discovering reimagined possibilities—more freedom and a deeper understanding of yourself.

A Powerful Path to Practice

You might be wondering, "What's next?" Maybe you feel energized and ready to continue, or perhaps you're questioning if this is enough. In a world that pushes "more is more," it's easy to doubt simplicity. But take a moment to reflect on the truth passed down by ancient wisdom: Less is more. By focusing on a few intentional poses, practiced mindfully, you create space for the magic of meaningful movement—proof that simplicity often leads to better outcomes.

Lasting progress—whether in movement, mindset, or lifestyle—comes from focusing on a few key practices and staying consistent. By mastering foundational movements first, you create a foundation for effective progress while staying safe and reducing the risk of strain or injury.

In this chapter, we'll explore why the 'less is more' approach works so well. Whether you're starting with the 7-Day Challenge or advancing to the 28-Day Challenge, you'll discover how gradual progress leads to meaningful, lifelong transformations.

The Power of Repetition

Remember the simple truths: Less is more, and small steps, repeated often, bring the best results. These aren't just catchy phrases—they're the foundation of a chair yoga practice that can change your life. Whether your goal is to relieve aches and pains or protect your quality of life, a steady, gentle approach is always the right one.

Sometimes, the simplest things in life have the greatest impact. Repetition is how you learn to ride a bike or remember the lyrics to your favorite song. Chair yoga works the same way. It doesn't need countless poses or complex choreography. Instead, it's about returning to a few carefully chosen movements and practicing them consistently. Because sometimes, the simplicity of repetition really is enough.

We designed your chair yoga plan to be easy to start—and even easier to sustain. This program includes built-in milestones to guide your progress. Each one builds on the last, creating a foundation that's both effective and lasting. Like any new skill, you start with the basics and practice until it feels natural. In the beginning, it's about getting it right. Over time, it becomes second nature. Eventually, every movement feels effortless—and that's where the real transformations begin.

A Lifestyle Worth Practicing

The 7-Day Challenge is the beginning of an exciting journey. But there's more. Beyond that, there are more phases to explore and even greater levels of wellness to discover. Each phase builds on the last, and every cycle deepens the benefits. Here's how to navigate your journey, one phase at a time:

1. **Begin with the 7-Day Challenge:** Follow the 5 daily routines for the first week, followed by 2 rest days. Practice each pose with care, paying attention to your body's signals.

2. **Transition to the 14-Day Challenge:** After completing the first week, move on to the next phase. Continue practicing the 5 daily routines, refining your movements and building confidence.

3. **Move to the 21-Day Challenge:** In the third week, deepen your practice by continuing the 5 daily routines. Give extra focus to breath and balance, and gently increase flexibility while honoring your body's limits.

4. **Advance to the 28-Day Challenge:** In the fourth week, practice the daily routines with greater intention and control. Gradually increase the intensity of each movement to improve mobility and strength.

5. **Integrate Chair Yoga into Daily Life:** After the 28-Day Challenge, revisit the routines with renewed confidence and perspective. The simplicity of repetition strengthens your mind-muscle connection, enhances mobility and flexibility, and relieves aches and pains—making mindful movement a way of life.

Remember, everyone's journey is unique. Make your practice personal by adapting it to your needs and celebrating your progress. If a phase gets interrupted, you can start over anytime—it's all part of the process. Honor your pace, and keep going—every step brings you closer to your goals. Who knows how far you can go? Now, let's explore how each stage supports your transformation.

The Magic of Mindful Movement

This journey is more than just a lifestyle change—it's life-changing. With mindful movement, subtle shifts grow into profound changes, proving that life is measured not in time but in the quality of each breath.

As you continue, the bond between body and mind grows stronger, bringing you closer to balance and well-being. Here's what you might experience along the way:

The 7-Day Challenge (Week 1): Reconnecting Mind and Body

In the first week, you'll notice a renewed sense of awareness. Gentle movements inspire curiosity about how your body feels and responds, uncovering subtle changes and insights you may have overlooked. Some poses build trust in your body's strength, while others remind you to move mindfully. This is a time for discovery and reconnection, deepening the bond between your body and mind.

The 14-Day Challenge (Week 2): Finding Focus and Confidence

In the second week, movements feel more familiar, and a sense of focus begins to grow. Confidence in your body's abilities deepens, bringing moments of gratitude, clarity, and a stronger connection to yourself. Building on the foundation of the first week, this phase helps you move with greater intention and trust.

The 21-Day Challenge (Week 3): Balancing Body and Mind

By the third week, a rhythm begins to emerge between your movements and thoughts. Strengthened mind-muscle connections make each movement more meaningful. Your body starts to move as one, guided by a clearer connection with your mind. A natural balance unfolds, revealing how even subtle movements are becoming more intentional and refined.

The 28-Day Challenge (Week 4): Redefining Reality

By week four, your movements feel purposeful, paired with a quiet confidence that extends beyond your practice. You may feel a renewed trust in your physical and emotional balance, along with growing confidence in your progress—bringing moments of clarity, energy, and the freedom to redefine your reality. Now, you're ready to embrace a new way of living—where mindful movement complements every aspect of an active life.

The Lifestyle Challenge (Beyond Week 4): A Life Without Limits

Beyond the 28-Day Challenge, chair yoga becomes more than just a routine—it's a natural part of an active lifestyle. The progress you've made reshapes your perspective and boosts your mood, supporting your well-being from the inside out. This is a time to embrace the strength, balance, and independence you've worked for, allowing mindful movement to make room for new beginnings. Each practice reconnects you with your purpose and helps you enjoy what matters most in life.

Mindful movement helps you rediscover your best self, revealing the potential within. As you reflect on your progress, remember: this is just the beginning. New possibilities may already be unfolding, and with each practice, you move closer to realizing your full potential.

Each day you commit to your practice strengthens the bond between body and mind—bringing lasting transformation, one breath at a time.

A Path to Possibilities

Whether you've already started your chair yoga journey or you're just beginning, you're not alone. Countless seniors have experienced the benefits of chair yoga—relief from stiffness, better mobility, improved flexibility, and more energy. These healing principles have been trusted for thousands of years, long before modern science confirmed how powerful they are. Here's what others are saying about their experience:

- "After my knee surgery, I was worried I'd never be able to walk comfortably again. But chair yoga helped me regain my strength and mobility. I never noticed how peaceful my walking path was until now; I can finally enjoy it without the aches and pains." - Robert, 68

- "I used to suffer from chronic back pain, but since I started practicing chair yoga, I've noticed a big improvement. The stretches and strengthening exercises have helped reduce my pain and improve my posture. I feel more comfortable and confident in my body again." - Sarah, 70

- "I was skeptical at first, but chair yoga has been a game-changer for my arthritis. The gentle movements have helped reduce the stiffness and pain in my joints. I'm able to move like I used to and enjoy my favorite hobbies without feeling anxious." - Bill, 65

- "This book has been a godsend for my aching joints. The chair yoga poses are so gentle, and they work. I have less pain! I feel more relaxed, more flexible, and not like a stranger in my own body." - Maria, 78

Chair yoga has already helped millions reclaim their mobility, reduce pain, and rediscover the freedom to move. With regular practice, you can discover the magic of mindful movement and the strength of simplicity—just like they did. So, what will your story be?

Namaste (nah-mah-stay)

"Namaste" is a traditional greeting that conveys respect and gratitude, recognizing our shared humanity. It connects us on a journey of growth and well-being.

In Sanskrit, "Namaste" is often translated as "I bow to you," but its meaning reaches beyond the literal. It acknowledges the goodness within each of us and reminds us that we are all connected. When we say "Namaste," we recognize the humanity within ourselves and others.

In chair yoga, "Namaste" holds a special significance. It reflects the rhythm of body and mind working together. Through each pose, you build not only physical strength and flexibility but also a sense of inner peace and balance. Your practice becomes a moment to honor your body, connect with yourself, and reflect with gratitude on your journey.

May the meaning of 'Namaste' guide you on your journey—a quiet reminder of the connection we all share. Let it inspire gratitude and compassion as you greet each day.

Namaste

Seniors Matter

Your journey matters. If this book has supported you in any way, please consider sharing your story with a review on **Amazon.com**. Your words could inspire someone to try chair yoga—and it just might change their life.

Together, we can make a difference. Because sometimes, change starts with something as simple as sharing your story.

My Chair Yoga Journey

Congratulations on reaching your final chair yoga journal entry! Take a moment to pause and reflect on how far you've come and what you've achieved. This is an accomplishment worth celebrating.

Use this space to note your favorite poses, the modifications that worked best, and any memorable moments from your practice. Let these notes remind you of your journey and inspire you to deepen your connection to body and mind through mindful movement.

Remember, this is just the beginning—it's your foundation for a life of freedom. May you discover the magic in mindful movement and the strength that comes from simplicity.

"Every mindful movement

brings balance to both

body and mind—

a path of promise

that blossoms

with every

daily practice."

—David Anthonie

Index

References

Bell, Baxter, and Nina Zolotow. *Yoga for Healthy Aging: A Guide to Lifelong Well-Being*. Boulder: Shambhala Publications, 2017.

Cheung, Catherine, et al. "Chair Yoga for Pain Management in Older Adults: A Pilot Study." *Journal of Pain Research* 12 (2019): 123-130.

Cramer, Holger, et al. "Yoga for Cardiovascular Health: A Systematic Review and Meta-analysis of Randomized Controlled Trials." *American Journal of Preventive Medicine* 49, no. 5 (2015): 753-764.

Dinardi, Michelle. *Chair Yoga for Seniors: A Complete Guide to Chair Yoga Poses and Sequences*. Ulysses Press, 2019.

Fishman, Loren M., and Carol Ardman. *Yoga for Arthritis: The Complete Guide*. New York: W.W. Norton & Company, 2008.

Fishman, Loren M., and Carol Ardman. *Yoga for Osteoporosis: The Complete Guide*. New York: W.W. Norton & Company, 2010.

Galantino, Mary Lou, et al. "Safety and Feasibility of Modified Chair Yoga on Functional Outcomes Among Elderly at Risk for Falls." *The Journals of Gerontology Series A: Biological Sciences and Medical Sciences* 67, no. 6 (2012): 648-655.

Garfinkel, Marian S., et al. "Yoga for Rheumatoid Arthritis: A Systematic Review." *Journal of Rheumatology* 33, no. 10 (2006): 2009-2017.

Garfinkel, M., et al. "Evaluation of a Yoga Based Regimen for Treatment of Osteoarthritis of the Hands." *Journal of Rheumatology* 27, no. 1 (2000): 234-238.

Hall, Amanda, et al. "Yoga for Chronic Neck Pain: A Systematic Review." *Clinical Rehabilitation* 30, no. 1 (2016): 4-11.

Khalsa, Sat Bir S. *Your Brain on Yoga: How Yoga Helps You Stay Calm, Sharp, and Happy*. New York: RosettaBooks, 2012.

Krucoff, Carol, Kristin Carson, and Marc Krucoff. "Relax into Yoga for Seniors: An Evidence-Informed Update for Enhancing Yoga Practice Benefits by Reducing Risk in a Uniquely Vulnerable Age Group." *OBM Geriatrics* 5, no. 1 (2021): 150.

Lasater, Judith Hanson. *Relax and Renew: Restful Yoga for Stressful Times.* Berkeley: Rodmell Press, 1995.

Long, Ray. *The Key Muscles of Yoga: Scientific Keys, Volume 1.* Little River, SC: Bandha Yoga Publications, 2006.

McCall, Timothy. *Yoga as Medicine: The Yogic Prescription for Health and Healing.* New York: Bantam Books, 2007.

Park, J., et al. "Chair Yoga: Benefits for Community-Dwelling Older Adults with Osteoarthritis." *Journal of Gerontological Nursing* 40, no. 10 (2014): 24-32.

Park, Jung Eun, et al. "A Pilot Randomized Controlled Trial of the Effects of Chair Yoga on Pain and Physical Function Among Community-Dwelling Older Adults with Lower Extremity Osteoarthritis." *Journal of Geriatric Physical Therapy* 39, no. 4 (2016): 168-177.

Ross, Alyson, and Sue Thomas. "The Health Benefits of Yoga and Exercise: A Review of Comparison Studies." *Journal of Alternative and Complementary Medicine* 16, no. 1 (2010): 3-12.

Saper, Robert B., et al. "Yoga for Chronic Low Back Pain in a Predominantly Minority Population: A Pilot Randomized Controlled Trial." *Alternative Therapies in Health and Medicine* 15, no. 6 (2009): 18-27.

Schaff, Nancy L. *Chair Yoga: Sit, Stretch, and Strengthen Your Way to a Happier, Healthier You.* Berkeley: Ulysses Press, 2020.

Sharma, Rajeev, et al. "Effect of a Single Session of Chair Yoga on Heart Rate Variability and Mood in Senior Citizens." *International Journal of Yoga* 9, no. 1 (2016): 32-37.

Sherman, Karen J., et al. "A Randomized Trial Comparing Yoga, Stretching, and a Self-care Book for Chronic Low Back Pain." *Archives of Internal Medicine* 171, no. 22 (2011): 2019-2026.

www.ingramcontent.com/pod-product-compliance
Lightning Source LLC
Chambersburg PA
CBHW081215260726
48653CB00010BA/3660